PROSTATE CANCER:

A DOCTOR'S

PERSONAL

TRIUMPH

PROSTATE CANCER:

A DOCTOR'S

PERSONAL

TRIUMPH

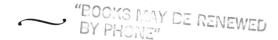

Saralee Fine and Robert Fine, M.D.

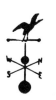

PAUL S. ERIKSSON, *PUBLISHER*
FOREST DALE, VERMONT

5 4 3 2 1

Library of Congress Cataloging-in-Publication Data

Fine, Robert, M.D.
Prostate cancer: a doctor's personal triumph / Saralee Fine and Robert Fine.
p.   cm.
Includes bibliographical references and index.
ISBN 0-8397-6808-7 (cloth)
1. Fine, Robert, M.D.—Health. 2. Prostate—Cancer—Patients—United States
Biography. 3. Radiologists—United States Biography.
RC280.P7F53   1999
326.1'9699463—dc21
[B]   99-22948
CIP

Design by Eugenie S. Delaney

For Dr. Haakon Ragde,
Kindness and Knowledge

ACKNOWLEDGMENTS

The authors thank Nycomed Amersham for their help with this book, Andrew Bright for his cooperation, the medical library at Emory University for its research capacity, Haakon Ragde for advice in medical editing and for his gift of self, Robert Meier who is as caring and gentle as it gets, Frank Manley for editorial assistance, Paula Vitaris for one zinger of an idea, Ivy Fischer Stone for friendliness, guidance, and tact, Paul and Peggy Eriksson for publishing and editing, and most of all our family and friends whose support sustained us during our ordeal.

Contents

〜

If you, that have grown old, were the first dead,
Neither catalpa tree nor scented lime
Should hear my living feet, nor would I tread
Where we wrought that shall break the teeth of Time.
Let the new faces play what tricks they will
In the old rooms; night can outbalance day,
Our shadows rove the garden gravel still,
The living seem more shadowy than they.

—WILLIAM BUTLER YEATS,
"THE NEW FACES"

Foreword

BY GORDON L. GRADO, M.D.

PROSTATE BRACHYTHERAPIST AND RADIATION ONCOLOGIST

One of my patients, who had done extensive research and reviewed all the treatment options, declared, "Prostate cancer is not a disease but a religion. As with any religion, it has its prophets and catechisms. Unfortunately, too often the religion followed is the one first met."

This applies to both physician and patient. Few physicians question their 'religion' except Dr. Haakon Ragde, who scrutinized the result of prostate-cancer treatments and sought out a better treatment option for his patients.

With the advent of improved diagnostic testing, the treatment of prostate cancer moved from one of the diagnosis of metastatic disease or locally advanced cancer to one of organ-confined disease. PSA, a blood test, and biopsy of the prostate with transrectal ultrasound led to earlier diagnosis and improved staging of prostate cancer.

PSA also provided the means of accurately assessing treatment results. It became more difficult to say, "we got it all," because the PSA could invalidate the procedure's success. All oncologists could now work to hone their skills. The playing field had changed as had the rules of the game. Results were now possible to assess accurately. Pathologists could better define the classification and extent of the disease, and radiologists were providing improved imaging modalities.

The end results of therapy are important to analyze but deal with more than just cure. Quality-of-life issues have achieved greater importance, as the patient assumes his rightful place in decision making. As a partner with his physician, the patient needs more information on results, side effects, and complications.

Prostate Cancer: A Doctor's Personal Triumph serves several valuable functions. It is a primer that leads the reader through the process of research, education, and decision making. It also demonstrates the need for a support network made up of those individuals important to the patient. These include his spouse, family, friends, and physicians. But most important is "to thine own self be true."

To search for and find answers, one must first define the questions. When consulting with physicians, patients are often deluged with answers for which they do not know the right questions. Therefore, the patient needs a handle on what issues should be addressed.

This book provides a chronology of the events that lead to treatment. The reader is able to go back or forward to reanalyze the issues, questions, and answers. Several physicians were consulted, and the reader can review the interactions and information as well as the workup and examination that precede treatment planning. One can also see the personal factors that the patient and family must consider and use to interpret the recommendations and forge *their* treatment program.

This book shows that one can indeed shape his care by interviewing, questioning, and identifying the strengths and weaknesses of the programs being evaluated. With many excellent treatments available, any given treatment needs to be questioned. Why is it recommended? What other approaches can be explored? What are the results? What are the side effects and complications? How are the treatment results being analyzed and updated? How does this program compare to others? Training is important. Experience essential. But technique defines the results.

Robert and Saralee Fine have opened up their lives, diagnosis, and decision making to others. They have explored their steps and slips, the conflicting information and recommendations, and have framed an approach that can help others. By researching and gaining the readily available knowledge to make an informed decision, they helped direct the construction of a viable and appropriate treatment program for them.

Their steps can help others by reducing the number of slips or hesitations. The mirror they hold up to the medical community and the patients' community can help both in the realistic analysis and expectations of treatment. This will eventually lead to and help answer questions regarding treatment—how much and when.

Introduction

by Harry R. Steele

Chairman, Canadian Airlines

C.E.O. and Chairman,

Newfoundland Capital Corporation, Limited

~

Prostate Cancer: A Doctor's Personal Triumph is an instructive book and should be read by anybody who has to make the difficult choice of how to deal with prostate cancer. When I was diagnosed with prostate cancer in December, 1996, I was shocked and bewildered but tried not to show it. I consulted the best surgeons I knew, and they all suggested radical surgery. I did not like what they told me. I spoke with men who had undergone radical surgery. I liked what they told me even less.

I had more or less been persuaded to have radical surgery and started taking hormones. I had been a vital person before, but those pills made me feel awful. They made me feel less manly and were the low point of my diagnostic phase.

A young doctor sensed my distress and gave me a magazine article, "Taking on Prostate Cancer," by Andy Grove, which renewed my hope. I called a doctor acquaintance of mine in Vancouver who had graduated from Johns Hopkins and discussed my dilemma. He said, "I will get in touch with the people at Johns Hopkins and call you back."

When he called, he put me in touch with Dr. Gerald Murphy at Pacific Northwest Cancer Foundation in Seattle. Dr. Murphy is a leading authority on prostate cancer. I had a candid conversation with him, and he reassured me. He spoke to me about Dr. Haakon Ragde.

Dr. Ragde called the next day, and we arranged an appointment in Seattle. On March 18, 1997, our oldest son, Peter, and I listened as Dr. Ragde went over the available options. After this meeting, there was no doubt whatsoever in my mind; I would proceed with seed implants.

Catherine, my wife of 42 years, Peter, and I returned to Seattle on May 11 and readied for the operation. My confidence was full. I cannot speak for Catherine and Peter. By now, I had come to really appreciate the whole Ragde team, including Donna and Kent.

I had my surgery late in the morning of May 13 and had recovered sufficiently by mid-afternoon for Dr. Ragde to drive me back to the motel. Dr. Ragde and his wife, Patricia, took us all to dinner—a truly memorable evening.

We visited the Ragde clinic the following day. It was only 24 hours since my surgery and, other than a little trouble urinating and some discomfort, all in all, good.

We flew to Halifax on May 15. I was back at work by 7:00 A.M. on the 16th. Since then, I have not missed a beat. I have checkups every six months and enjoy perfect health. All functions normal.

In retrospect, being diagnosed with prostate cancer has been the most traumatic experience of my life. Nobody could tell me exactly what to do, and I understand why. We looked at all the options and had to ignore some strong, well-intentioned advice. I am glad we did. When one reaches seventy you realize nothing is forever, but the road ahead looks okay to me.

Prostate Cancer: A Doctor's Personal Triumph will help anybody who has to deal with the disease. If this book had been available to me, it would have saved so much anguish and made our decision much more timely and easier. Saralee and Dr. Robert, thanks for a great effort and a good read. You have shown how to handle a difficult situation well.

PROSTATE CANCER:

A DOCTOR'S

PERSONAL

TRIUMPH

Discovery

~

SARALEE

SATURDAY, AUGUST 30, 1997

I keep hitting wrong keys on my computer, because I'm shaking. The result is a worse hodge-podge than usual. The delete button is working hard. It's 11:30 A.M., and I'm already drinking wine. Yesterday we learned that Bob has cancer of the prostate gland.

That morning, I fed Praise, our Siamese kitten, worked out on our exercise machine, and watered all my plants. I stroked Praise, snuggled beside me in bed, as I read Salman Rushdie's incredible and dense prose. Hours and hours of quiet luxury and peace of mind that I may never find again.

When the phone rang about 3 o'clock, I realized it had rung for the first time that day. I picked up the receiver, and a woman said, "May I speak to Dr. Fine?"

"He's not here. This is Mrs. Fine. How may I help you?" I said.

"Can I reach him at his office?"

"No, he probably left his office about 2 and is driving home now. Would you care to leave a message?"

"No. We'll be here until 4:30 or 5. Have him call his urologist when he gets home."

Bob's urologist had done an ultrasound exam and a biopsy of his prostate gland on Monday. The receptionist's refusal to leave a message saying that the test results had been normal was a bad sign. I was too anxious to read any more.

An ultrasound exam is a study using sound waves to penetrate the body and evaluate tissue anatomy. The patient feels nothing. A wand is moved over whatever area is to be studied. Bob does ultrasound exams frequently.

Bob had told me that an ultrasound of the prostate gland is more involved. Because the gland is housed deep within the pelvis, the wand needs to be placed in the rectum. There, it will be right up against the gland, and the pictures will be good.

That sounded painful. My gynecologist had recently examined me. To feel the shape and tilt of my uterus, she had simultaneously placed a finger in my vagina and another up my rectum. The end of my anus had felt swollen for days.

For the biopsy, the urologist had taken slivers of tissue removed from Bob's prostate gland and sent them to a hospital, so a pathologist could see if any cancer was present. Neither of us had expected that the urologist would biopsy Bob.

I had asked Bob to let me go with him for the ultrasound. He said no. It would be the last time he'd go to a doctor alone. He deserved and would get all my comfort and support.

I got back into bed and wished Bob home. When he arrived the telephone rang. It was his radiology tech with an emergency exam for him to read on his tele-radiology. This computer setup sends films from his hospital, ninety miles away, and enables him to read emergency exams on the screen beside his desk.

I had almost called Bob earlier. It was the Friday before Labor Day, and he'd want to check with his urologist to see if his biopsy results were back. Otherwise, we wouldn't know until Tuesday. But I didn't call him. Neither of us anticipated abnormal results.

Bob's universal good health during our forty-year marriage has made us come to take his well-being for granted. We both knew the ultrasound had proved normal. The biopsy had been thrown in for completeness.

Bob turned on the tele-radiology in his library and called his urologist. I was in the kitchen when he called to me. I walked into his study. He was hanging up the telephone.

"Saralee," he said, "my urologist says the biopsy is positive. I have cancer of the prostate."

Instinctively, we reached out to one another and held each other close, hugging. We didn't say anything. We were incredulous, not believing what we'd been told. In shock.

"I think my doctor was surprised, too," Bob said, "but his last words were 'with treatment, you will be cured'."

Bob and I repeated "you will be cured" over and over again, a mantra to get us through the endless holiday weekend. With that, he turned, walked to his desk, and read the exam that had arrived on his computer screen. I was amazed at his self-control.

BOB

Before a routine physical exam with my internist six years ago, I had blood work done at the country hospital where I practice radiology. My chief tech suggested that a routine PSA, a prostate specific antigen study, be included, because I was almost sixty.

A PSA exam, done from a blood sample, measures what's given off by both the normal prostate and by cancerous tissues of the prostate. Little antigen escapes from a healthy gland, so an elevated PSA is a possible danger signal of prostate cancer.

My PSA result was 2.0, and the normal range is anything less than 4.0. My internist found my prostate gland enlarged during a digital rectal exam, but that is normal in a man my age.

In March of 1996, another blood test was done in preparation for a physical exam, and the PSA result was 2.2. My internist and I agreed that this minimal increase was to be expected along with the enlarging of the prostate gland with age. Neither of us thought much about that then.

Blood tests were done in preparation for my routine physical exam this month. These showed a few red blood cells in my urine, insignificant, and my prostate specific antigen at 3.7.

I was worried about the sudden rise in my PSA, but I didn't want to scare Saralee. So I told her nothing.

"You'll be fine. You always are," Saralee said as we drank mugs of my hazelnut coffee in bed and read the newspaper on Thursday, the morning of my physical.

"I hope so, but my PSA has jumped from 2.2 to 3.7 in sixteen months," I said.

"How long have you known that?"

"Since my blood results came back. About a week."

"Why didn't you tell me?"

"I couldn't see any point in both of us worrying about a test that's still within normal range."

My internist did not examine me that day. He called a urologist instead, told him about the jump in my PSA, and made an appointment for me to have an ultrasound exam the following Monday morning. Then we sat in his office and talked, mostly about investments and retirement. We've both been threatening to retire, and we both keep putting it off just a little while longer.

I gave myself an enema on Monday morning in preparation for the ultrasound. Just after 10 o'clock, I was sitting on the urologist's examining table sans shoes, trousers, and underpants. I covered my privates with a disposable waterproof sheet. When the door opened, a man in surgical scrubs entered, smiled, and shook hands with me.

"Bob, you've come to the right man. Prostate cancer runs in my family. Though I'm not fifty yet and my PSA is normal, I'm going to have an ultrasound done soon, just to be extra sure."

"How long does this exam take?"

"About five minutes," he said. "And I'll be as gentle as possible."

I winced.

"Please turn on your left side and bend your knees toward your chest."

I did that, and he examined me first with his finger.

"So far so good," he said. "No nodules I can palpate."

A nodule is a localized area of enlargement that can be felt. It increases the likelihood of malignancy.

"Now I'm going to do the ultrasound study."

He tried to insert the ultrasound probe into my rectum, but my sphincter was too tight.

"Relax," he said, "and I'll put more lubricant on the probe."

I tried hard to relax, and he was successful in sliding the tube far up my rectum to envision my prostate gland. As he did the study, he rotated and angled the probe. I stiffened my neck muscles and clutched the examining table edge. Five minutes had never seemed so long.

"I don't see any obvious abnormal echoes," he said, "but there are a few dark areas. I want to do a needle biopsy."

The biopsy seemed superfluous.

"What will it feel like?"

"Like a pin prick."

"How many pin pricks?"

"About six, but don't hold me to an exact number. They make a loud sound, so I'll warn you by counting backwards—3, 2, 1— and then I'll do a biopsy. Three, two, one."

'Bang.' He was right about the noise, but the pin pricks were punches jammed deep inside me. The pain reverberated down through my balls. He repeated the process five more times. I was exhausted when he finished, as much from the stress as from the pain.

"We'll call you when the biopsy results have gone through the lab. It's usual to do a PSA exam every six months, but I prefer having it done every four months," he said.

I was relieved. If he was talking about routine PSAs, I was far from cancer.

I cleaned myself up from the lubricant and blood. I stuffed tissues between my rectum and underwear, so I wouldn't stain my clothes. The receptionist handed me some capsules and a sheet of directions on the way out. I shuffled out of the office and walked gingerly to my car.

There, I read the directions, divided into three sections. Under things not to do for 24 hours were strenuous physical activity, sex, and straining while moving my bowels. The thought of needing to move my bowels was unnerving.

Under what to expect was blood in the rectum, in urine, and in semen. Under problems to call about were excessive bleeding or clots in urine or stool, difficulties in voiding, and chills or fever over 101 degrees.

The capsules were Floxin, a state-of-the-art antibiotic. If I still hurt or felt a burning sensation while urinating after taking them for 3 days, I had an infection and needed more Floxin.

Saralee had asked to come with me that morning, but I refused. My brother, Howard, had this exam done several years before, and he claimed it was nothing. I wished I had taken her with me. Saralee would have driven me home. She would have comforted me.

She was waiting for me when I got home.

"You look pale" she said.

I handed her the sheet of directions.

She read it and said, "How bad do you hurt?"

"Enough to cancel any errands you might have in mind and sit quietly at a movie this afternoon."

The pain continued through the day. We went to sleep early, and

I felt decent by the next morning.

I work on Tuesday and Wednesday mornings. I had a bridge game scheduled for Tuesday afternoon and would do my billings that evening. I sleep at a motel on Tuesday nights to minimize my ninety mile drive on the Interstate to and from Atlanta.

SARALEE

I sat on Bob's plaid sofa as he read the emergency CT scan after he talked with his urologist that Friday, and we learned that he had cancer. He seemed calm, efficient, and professional.

A CT scan, properly called a computerized axial tomography scan, is a circular series of X-rays taken by a machine that goes around the body. A computer puts the pictures together, generating images that are like slices of anatomy.

"What happens now?" I said when Bob had finished calling in the report to his hospital.

"We're both going to meet with my urologist at 4:30 next Wednesday. He says that by the time we've finished talking, we'll both know as much as any internist about cancer of the prostate."

"Isn't he at his office now?"

"Yes."

"Call him back. Let's drive there and see him right away."

Bob called, but the receptionist told him his urologist was leaving to do surgery. Wednesday at 4:30 was the earliest time he could meet us. I felt hostile toward this urologist.

It is not unusual for me to view doctors with animosity. I have lupus which took years to diagnose. I encountered plenty of doctors along the way. Most of them viewed me as an interesting object. I wanted to be a subject, subjected to a cure. Most of them gave up on me fast when they couldn't figure out what was wrong.

"If your urologist is so busy, who can we talk to?" I asked.

We sat thinking, until I realized that we knew a radiotherapist, a horseback riding buddy of years past. Because he was a class act as a person, I anticipated he'd be the same as a physician.

Bob began looking through the yellow pages but had trouble finding a listing of therapeutic radiologists, those physicians who treat cancer with radiation. I grabbed the business directory. We found the radiotherapist's number simultaneously.

I sat on Bob's sofa and listened as they talked. Afterwards, Bob told me what he had said.

"He told me that cancer of the prostate can be treated with surgery, radiation therapy, or both."

"What's his advice?"

"He recommends radiation therapy, because the surgery is so radical. Not only is the prostate removed, but much of the adjacent area as well."

"Why?"

"To get rid of any lymph nodes that may be cancerous as well. Radiation has the same wide-spread effect of deadening the prostate and adjacent lymph nodes without radical surgery."

"If it's so wide-spread, what else does it take away?"

"Good question. I'll research that in my radiology journals."

"I'll write about how miserable we feel."

BOB

We called our daughters that first night. Wendy, our computer whiz, advised me to use the Internet as a research tool. She kept crying and saying "Daddy, I love you so much" over and over again. She made me cry with her.

Jody, our clinical psychologist, told us to get into bed and hug a lot. We followed her advice. During that dark night, our two warm bodies curled comfortingly together like spoons.

I called my brother Howard who told me that every man gets prostate cancer if he lives long enough. Cancer of the prostate is an inevitable by-product of old age. He advised caution in treatment.

I read medical journals that endless weekend, and Saralee wrote on our computer. Busy work to make the time pass until we could meet with the urologist.

I began a compulsive folder of my PSA results augmented by edited comments based on what I'd read. I bored Saralee with endless specifics. I would learn later that these facts I'd read were outdated, but nothing could curb my zeal in amassing them. I compiled data like the coin collection of my boyhood. Yes, I was panicky.

She was panicky, too. She agreed to let me do whatever I felt was beneficial, any procedure I felt would make me comfortable.

"It's your cancer," she said, "and our lives."

Then, one of us remembered we had planned a fortieth anniversary gift to share; we were going to Italy in October. That trip got put on permanent hold.

My life was at stake.

SARALEE

During the weekend, I remembered that my cousin Larry in California was a medical oncologist, a doctor who treats cancer patients. The three of us talked by phone. What I learned made me decide to monitor as many of Bob's phone conversations as I could.

"Don't do surgery," he told Bob. "Your prostate is buried deep behind a mass of bones and is impossible to reach. The procedure is bloody and none too discrete."

"But with surgery, my prostate will be gone."

"The post-surgical complications are a nightmare. Choose something less radical. I put my patients on Lupron immediately."

"What's that?" Bob asked.

"Cancer of the prostate depends on testosterone for growth. Lupron lowers testosterone."

"What are its side effects?"

"Lupron lowers libido."

"Libido, as in sex drive?" I asked.

"Yes."

"Thanks, but no thanks," I said. "Sex is one of the great things we've got going for us."

"We want to keep sex in our lives forever," Bob agreed.

We were already aware our days as sexual partners could be ended by any treatment Bob chose.

BOB

I met Saralee the spring she graduated from high school, just before I began medical school. At a friend's house, I was looking at the latest copy of my high school yearbook. I was bored with everyone I was dating and looking for someone new.

I saw her photograph and said, "Who's that? She's sure a looker."

"I don't know. Maybe my sister does."

His sister knew Saralee and introduced us by telephone. Saralee agreed to meet me that afternoon. I dressed in a blue oxford cloth button-down with my monogram embroidered on the pocket and properly scruffy saddle shoes. She must have found me appealing, because she accepted a date for that evening.

While we talked and began learning about one another, the telephone rang.

Her grandmother answered the phone and said, "It's your parents."

"What do they want?" Saralee asked.

"To tell you they'll be late and won't be taking you to dinner."

Saralee shrugged.

"You'd better get here sometime soon," Grandma said to them. "The man who will marry your daughter is sitting beside her on your sofa."

That was clever intuition on her part.

We dated steadily for the next several weeks, until I left for a cross-country tour of the forty-eight states with a friend. We took my car, a Chevy convertible that needed a quart of oil every hundred miles. We bought oil by the case. The trip was one last fling before the rigors of medical school.

I wrote Saralee some letters, not exactly love letters. Mostly, I described what I was seeing. I usually told her "I miss you" at the end. She still has those letters, tied with a faded blue ribbon. I called her when we reached California.

On the way back to Pittsburgh, we stopped at Phoenix. I visited the fiancée of a good friend.

"I've met the girl I love," I confided to her. "Can you help me choose a gift for her?"

"Sure," she said and chose a bottle of cologne for me.

Soon after I got back from my trip, Saralee stopped dating anyone else. She told me that other men made her uncomfortable. She felt on stage and obliged to make endless small talk. With me, she could talk or be silent. She felt comfortable with me. We both knew that we already belonged to each other.

Many couples who meet and marry young grow apart as they mature. They divorce. We were lucky. During our forty-some-year relationship, we grew closer. We depend on one another even more now, as we approach old age.

Since I sleep at a motel on Tuesday, Saralee and I reunite with glee every Wednesday afternoon, as if we'd been apart for weeks. We fall into bed together to make glorious and horny love. Afterwards, we nap and shower; then, we fix dinner together.

SARALEE

As we hugged in bed one afternoon that endless Labor Day weekend, Bob said, "I'm afraid to move. I might be metastasizing."

"What's that mean?" I asked.

"It means I could be spreading cancer cells all over my body."

I sat up in bed, pointed at the ski machine we had exercised on earlier, and said, "Did you think you were metastasizing when you worked out this morning?"

"No."

"Then you're probably not spreading any cancer around now either."

"I'm a mess," he said and came close to crying.

"You're definitely not a mess. You're dealing with a new concept. Mortality. It takes a while to adjust."

"Yes. It stinks."

"Definitely. Foul black stench of death. But we've smelt it before."

"When?"

"Ages ago. Fifteen, maybe twenty years ago. When we found out I had lupus, and it could kill me."

"Yes. I haven't thought about your dying from lupus for years."

"I remember begging you to cut back on your practice, so we could travel more."

"That's true."

When lupus attacks the organs—kidneys, liver, heart, brain— any of the vital organs, it destroys the membrane that surrounds each organ. Without the protective membrane, the organ begins to deteriorate and eventually can no longer function.

"Look, we got so comfortable with the stench of lupus, we can't smell it anymore."

"I guess so."

"My grandma used to say that if you hang long enough, you'll get used to hanging. We'll adapt."

"Lupus isn't cancer. The word cancer conjures fear."

I had no consoling answer for that, so I hugged him. I tried hard not to cry. I didn't want my fear to make his cancer more difficult. A couple of times in the middle of the night, I woke up wailing, way out of control. He'd wake, too, and hold me in his comforting arms.

Once, tears came rolling down my face as we walked our miles together. I hoped he didn't notice, or, if he did, he thought the wind had made my eyes water. We walk four miles in an hour. Exercise is especially important for us now. A fabulous way of lowering stress. Some days, I'm so scared that my knees shake. Then, I can hardly keep up our pace.

My cousin called again on Sunday morning to extol the virtues of Lupron. Bob answered the phone, on his side of the bed, and handled the call. We were reading *The New York Times* in bed and drinking coffee. Both of us had temporarily forgotten about cancer. I wished my cousin hadn't reminded us.

Bob is so much more rational than I, so cool and controlled. What does he feel beneath that impeccable exterior?

BOB

I felt horrible, and Saralee was hounding me to tape-record emotions that I wanted to hide. I use a recorder for my X-ray dictations, and she uses it as a writer's tool. We fooled around for a while comparing tape recorder techniques. Our hands were none too steady. The shaking recorder expressed our emotions.

We sat in her library with its computer desk and her grandmother's desk where she does any business I can con her into doing. I sat on a bentwood rocker, while she sprawled on her sofa. She set the recorder beside me on a drop-leaf table.

"Testing, 2, 4, 6, 8, who do we appreciate?" I said.

"Please forget all about being taped," she said and moved the recorder to a table between us. "We'll have a normal conversation."

I wondered how any conversation about cancer could be considered normal.

"The most comforting words I've heard were my urologist's. He said, 'the worst scenario is that after you are treated you will be cured.'"

Minimize, I thought. Keep the mood light. If you let her know how frightened you are, you'll both collapse in a pool of tears. I must stay cool and figure out how to deal with this.

"Even though cancer of the prostate is known to be a disease of older men, I never thought of myself as older."

"Because you don't act like an old man. You're very active."

"Here I am."

"Yes. And here I am, right beside you. I'd do anything to make this easy for you."

I stood up, afraid to give vent to my emotions. We took a break. I made myself a sandwich and fed her a bite. We each drank a glass of wine. Then, we began recording again. She kept bugging me to tell her how I felt about having cancer.

"When I hit 65, I did have a big emotional hit, " I said. "Now, I know I'm vulnerable."

I stuttered over the word vulnerable. I hoped she didn't notice, because I needed to control my emotions and think rationally. I needed to control her emotions, too. We mustn't break down.

"Why did I get this blood test early? Am I fixated on my anus, prostate, and penis?"

This was a banal assessment of myself, meant to lead us away from carcinoma, a concept we were both finding difficult to confront.

"Of course not," she said.

"I felt I should have a physical exam and blood work-up every two years. Fortunately, I didn't wait two years. That was not just luck.

It was very skillful."

I might as well give myself a little credit. It made the messiness of what lay ahead more tolerable.

I wanted a rational mind-set for her. Intellectual. Thought through. Prepared. Nothing like the terror I felt now.

"But I should have remembered that I had my blood work and physical exam done by my birthday, at the end of January. This time it was six months before my birthday. Very fortunate."

"Yes, fortunate."

I wanted Saralee to see the problem in its best light. That it was good to have discovered this early. I wanted to convince myself of this as well.

"Now that I have this diagnosis, I'm looking forward to talking with the urologist on Wednesday. I know he will be encouraging."

I was dreading the discussion, too. Saralee's cousin and our radiotherapist friend had both warned me about the dangers and complications of surgery.

"We'll start to get the program planned and get the treatment going," I said. "We'll have to decide when the treatment starts."

"You'll have to decide."

"When I have something to do, I like to do it immediately."

"That's you."

We were drinking much more wine than usual. Saralee claimed they were making the bottles smaller.

"Do you hurt at all when you move?" she asked.

"Not a bit. But I'm slower and more conscious of how I move, probably because of all the wine we drink."

It would hardly do to tell her I felt myself destructing with every wary step I took.

"Okay, so you feel your body is fragile."

"Of course it's fragile. The ass area is fragile."

She laughed out loud. I made her find something humorous

about my rectal exam and the residual blood in my urine and semen. Her laughter cheered and comforted me.

"The rest of me is not fragile," I assured her. "I'm in very very good shape."

That was daytime talk. Everything was more frightening at night.

"I dread the results of the acid phosphatase test and the MRI exam."

An acid phosphatase exam is a blood test to determine bone metastasis. Whether the cancer has spread into surrounding bone.

MRI stands for magnetic resonance imaging. It gives a three-dimensional scan of the body. Like a CT scan, an MRI produces images that are like slices of the anatomy.

"My brother, Howard, had an MRI. He said being in the tube gave him claustrophobia."

"I remember his saying that."

"I don't expect either of these tests to be positive. But you want to deny, you want to hide from tests. Because of any slight chance they might prove positive."

"Yes, I understand."

"I'm beginning to realize knowledge is not necessarily beneficial."

That was both true and false. My intellect demanded information. My emotions despised it.

"And my PSA is low. Chances should be wonderful."

I desperately wanted this to be true.

"Typically, I know it's a slow growing cancer—except in some cases. And in the worst scenario, even if it's not cured, it'll be many years until I succumb."

Hogwash. I wanted it cured, all cured, definitely cured. With no threat left hanging over me.

"Fortunately, I have you to share life with. I'll grill a steak for us tonight. My biggest worry is whether I'll get it done right."

Saralee chuckled. She likes hers rare, and I like mine medium rare. We share a steak by giving her the less cooked center and me the crisp ends.

"Let's worry about which wine we should have with the steak."

SARALEE

It takes extra effort to grill outdoors when you live in an apartment building, but a charred sirloin is worth the work. Bob went downstairs and lit coals on our hibachi, then he came back up. I opened wine and fixed a salad—greens and a tomato he had grown.

When we thought the coals were hot enough, we went downstairs together. We rarely grill out anymore. It takes two elevators to get to our cook-out site, the public pavement. Grilling is prohibited on our condominium grounds.

We sat on wood planks that bordered the garden next door and watched the steak sizzle. When we agreed it was done, Bob carried our prize through the garage and onto the elevator that took us to the lobby. We crossed the lobby; our desk attendant sniffed approvingly. A young woman on the elevator asked if we wanted help eating dinner.

I had eaten little since Friday. The bad news had stolen my appetite. Tonight, we both ate with gusto and dunked crusty bread chunks in the steak's juice.

"Bob," I said, "do you remember my going to a psychologist when we planned Wendy's wedding at the farm?"

"Yes. You didn't want a farm wedding. You wanted it in Washington D.C."

"That seemed logical. They both live there. Ralph since birth, Wendy for over ten years. I thought none of their Washington friends would come to our isolated farm, and few family members would show up either."

"Yes."

"You insisted on personally grooming our acreage. I thought you'd kill yourself, and there'd be nobody to give the bride away."

"You were wrong about that."

"Yes. It was a wonderful wedding. Tons of people showed up. They thought the farm was a super setting for a wedding."

"Wendy and Ralph did, too. They thank us whenever they go to anybody else's wedding and on every anniversary."

"Anyhow, the psychologist told me to put together a support team. People I could talk with when I got anxious."

"You did that."

"It helped. I think we need a support team now. Not a big team. Just a few friends who will listen to our dilemma and comfort us."

"I don't know. We'd have to keep it small. I don't want many people to know anything about this. I need my disease to stay private."

"I know about your sense of privacy. I'll respect that."

"People don't want to talk about cancer. They want to talk about happy things. After a while, illness cancels a relationship."

"A few special friends will want to help. Your internist's wife has called to say they'll do anything to ease us through this. She ended with 'I love you.'"

"Keep it small. Cancer is so ominous. I wonder if friends will think shaking my hand, hugging me, or kissing me may contaminate them."

"That's crazy. Let's call Piera and Addison and tell them."

They live four floors from us. We've shared many good times together. When Piera and I have problems with our daughters, we share that, too. I knew they'd relate.

Our doorbell rang in half an hour. Bob opened the door, and Ad wrapped both arms around him in a bear hug. Piera kissed him. So much for his contamination theory.

We sat in our living room, as we normally did with nibbles

before going out for dinner. Ad sat beside me; and Piera, beside Bob. To say that they were sympathetic would be British understatement. We were blanketed in the warmth of their support.

"We want to put together a small support team to help us," I said.

"We're honored to be included," Ad said.

"Thanks," Bob said. "We'll try not to be a burden."

"On the contrary, we want you to lean on us. We'll be here for you when you need us."

The next day was Monday, Labor Day. We drank coffee in bed and read *The Atlanta Journal-Constitution*, loaded with sale ads. Neither of us wanted to shop. We couldn't find a decent movie either. We had a bad case of the blahs. Maybe we'd stay in bed all day.

"I've run out of journal articles," Bob said. "I need more prostate-cancer information. So I can decide what treatment to have. I need recent information."

"We researched together at Emory University's medical library when I started menopause. It's a super medical library. I'll bet they have the latest cancer journals."

"Good idea. I can find current information there. Articles that have just been published and focus on my problem."

We went together. Bob did research and xeroxed pertinent information. He created a list of articles to be read by using the authors' names and the bibliography at the end of each article he read. He seemed stimulated by what he was learning. More in control. Less of a victim.

I sat quietly, a mute spectator. I tried to concentrate on Salman Rushdie's literary style but found myself more concerned about Bob Fine.

After a few hours of intense research, he said, "I've had as much information as I can handle for today."

We returned to the medical library frequently. It became a focal point in his education and eventual ability to make a decision that might work for him.

Late that afternoon, we called Mark and Judith. They are relatively new friends; Mark and Bob respect each other's minds, and Judith and I could have been hatched from the same egg. They weren't at home. We left a message on their voice mail that asked them to call us.

We also called John and Nancy in Denver. We've remained close friends since we all lived in Milwaukee more than twenty years ago. Our first spring, we planted a perennial garden in our side yard beside their house. We dug the bed, smashed clods of earth into fine soil, added fertilizer, and planted the flowers. It's the blue delphiniums I remember best. The project lasted all weekend.

On that Sunday afternoon, John crossed from their lawn to ours. He carried a tray in his hands. On it were an icy pitcher and frosty glasses.

"You look like you need a break. Shall we drink martinis?"

We promptly christened our project "the martini garden" It was the start of a great friendship.

John and Nancy weren't at home, so I left a message. John had dealt with prostate cancer. His voice on their recorder was both calm and congenial.

"John," I said, "hearing your voice is reassuring. Bob has prostate cancer. We need your help. Please call when you can. Love from both of us."

On Tuesday morning, Bob left for his hospital. On Tuesday morning, I learned how to cry. Judith returned our call.

"What are you doing?" she asked.

"Crying. Can't you tell?"

"Saralee, what's wrong?"

"Bob has prostate cancer, and I don't want to cry in front of him. He's not crying, and I know he wants no tears from me."

"Then you have plenty of reason to cry. I want to help you as much as I can."

"I don't think anyone can help us until 4:30 on Wednesday. We'll meet with the urologist who diagnosed Bob's cancer, and he'll explain what to do."

"Let's have dinner together soon."

"Okay, but Dutch treat, like we always do."

Bob didn't want people to think of him as disabled, to pity or shun him. Judith instinctively picked up on how he felt.

"Dutch treat, it will be."

We set a date for dinner.

I'd like to say I exercised on that Tuesday and Wednesday, but I probably didn't. I'd like to claim I wrote on Tuesday and Wednesday, but I certainly didn't. I frequently write for six or eight hours at a stretch, often more. The two days when I'm alone are normally my productive writing corridor.

Nothing felt normal anymore. I couldn't even read. I spent protracted periods in my closet, curled like a fetus, hidden and howling.

Alternatives

~

BOB

We arrived at my urologist's office at 4:30 on Wednesday afternoon. We sat for a while in his waiting room, not because he wanted to put us off. He wanted our appointment to be the last of the day, so he could tell us everything we needed to know. When the time came, he met with us in his office. He was dressed in green surgical scrubs.

"Do you mind if I record this?" Saralee asked and held up her tape recorder. "Sometimes we remember different things."

"Sure, if you want to," he said. "Why don't you two sit with me on the sofa?"

He sat between us, a companionable bulk, green clad. Robin Hood servicing the truly poor.

"I'm going to get a legal pad and walk you through the whole thing."

"Okay," I said. "Thanks."

He settled between us.

"We've got three legal pads, one for each of us," I said and laughed nervously.

"That's fine. Basically, if you did not have PSA, you would not know you had anything wrong."

That was fortunate.

"Okay. And when you stage a prostate cancer in the U. S., we use A, B, C, D. Stage A cancers are found after a TURP."

A TURP is a transurethral resection of the prostate. Going through the urethra, the surgeon cuts away a portion of the enlarged prostate gland. This allows the man to urinate more easily, because his smaller prostate doesn't block his bladder.

"Saralee doesn't know what all of this means or that I haven't had a TURP."

"Right. The PSA is normal, the rectal exam is normal, but one in ten men will be found to have spots of cancer."

"What he's saying," I explained to her, "is that you find cancer in people you don't even suspect it in."

"Now, there's a new way of staging called increased PSA. Remember the TNM classification you had to memorize in med school?"

"I haven't thought about it since then."

TNM means tumor nodes metastases. The TNM classification shows how far advanced a tumor is, the aggressiveness of the tumor itself, and whether it has metastasized or not. Metastases refer to tumor that has spread beyond the prostate gland.

He drew a graph and said, "In a TNM classification, yours would be a T1c, and this would be a T2, meaning a nodule felt rectally. T1a and b are diagnoses made by pathologists on prostate specimens. A T1c is diagnosed by biopsy, prompted perhaps by an increase in PSA velocity or an abnormality on transrectal ultrasound. Okay?"

"Okay," I said, but I was confused by his rapid explanation of prostate cancer classification.

"So that would be your stage, a T1c based on PSA change."

I didn't dare look across at Saralee to see how confused or scared all this medical gobble-de-goop was making her. I needed to deal with the facts.

"A B1 or T2a has a little mini-nodule. A B2 or T2b has a bigger nodule on one side, and a B3 or T2c has cancer on both sides."

A nodule one can feel indicates the probability of tumor.

"So he's right here," Saralee said and pointed to a place on the graph he had drawn.

"He's right there," the urologist answered her. "We'll put a little star by him. That's you."

"All right. I'm T1c," I said.

"T1c. I prefer a TPSA or an increased PSA only. They're all the same."

TPSA, a misnomer, also refers to tumor with an elevated PSA. The PSA can be below 4, which is still normal. Mine was 3.7.

"You can draw a line," he said. "Everything above the line is curable by surgery. Below the line it's not. You're far above the line, so you have options of radiation up here, too."

"Right."

"Below the line there is no other option but surgery. In a stage C gland, the cancer has broken outside of the capsule but has not gone anywhere else in the same general area. Radiation is your only chance to cure that. A D1 gland, the cancer has gone to lymph nodes."

The body has a lymphatic system, a roadway for lymph to travel along. Lymph nodes are stations along the way that cancer can invade and enlarge. With D1, the cancer has already spread outside the prostate gland to lymph nodes in the pelvis.

"A D2 gland, the cancer has gone to bone."

With D2, the cancer has traveled to both the nodes and the surrounding bones, particularly those of the pelvic arch.

"And the grade of tumor. He's calling it a Gleason 6, but he doesn't really have much data to go on. He's calling it a 3 plus 3, but basically, you've got a 1 millimeter focus in 1 core of the 6 I took."

"How big is a core?"

"A few millimeters wide."

A millimeter is about the width of a piece of dental floss. It's minuscule. I was darn lucky he had found the cancer in my prostate.

"Did you sample a variety of sites?"

"Of course. With that, everything falls out on a bell curve. You get Gleason grading."

Gleason grading was what the pathologist had called a 6 in my case, a 3 plus 3. It's a way of grading the cancer by looking through a microscope at slides showing tissue taken for biopsy.

"They take an area of most differentiated tumor and an area of least differentiated tumor and tie them together. So the score goes from two to ten," the urologist said.

The degree of differentiation translates into the aggressiveness of the cancer cells.

"Oh, there's not a '1'," I said and laughed.

"No 1. 1 plus 1. You can't get any lower than 2."

"I understand."

"Okay. So before we had Gleason score, we called it well differentiated, moderately differentiated, and poorly. Just like the word says, you don't want poor in anything."

"Uh huh."

"Gleason 9 and 10's are almost always spread when you find them. Gleason 2, 3, and 4's are almost never spread when you find them. You're sitting right here in the middle with a low volume tumor."

He pointed to 6 on the Gleason score. Low volume meant a small area of cancer involvement.

"Yes."

"That's more good news. It's hard to tell somebody that over the phone."

"This was a terrible weekend."

"I know."

"I wish you had told me how little the area of involvement was.

We would have both been less anxious."

"Yes. Here's where your internist did a great job. PSA less than 10. Depending on who you read, 80% or 85% of these are self-confined."

Self-confined means that the cancer has not spread outside the prostate gland.

"Your numbers should be better than that. They should be closer to 100. We had such a hard time finding it."

"Good," I said.

"In a PSA greater than 10, there's a 60% positive margin rate."

After the surgeon has removed the whole prostate gland, a pathologist studies it. Of particular interest is the margin, the periphery or edge of the gland. If the cancer has penetrated the margin, it is likely that there is cancer outside of the gland, too.

"Even with that, we'll cure a lot of those guys. Okay? So you're in a favorable category of beating this thing and living out your own life span."

"Yes."

"You look at disease-free survival, and the study I'm going to show you is the only prospective study that we have published."

A prospective study takes a current group of people and follows them for a period of time in the future.

"Okay."

"It drives the radiation guys crazy. It was done in the Duke VA system by a guy named Paulson. It's the only prospective study we've got published, and the survival curve pretty much mimics the survival curve of normal survival."

"That would be with surgery?"

"External beam is fine for the first while, then it slowly comes down."

External beam radiation is X-radiation aimed at a tumor in the body with the intent of shrinking or completely killing cancer cells. Tumor cells are more sensitive to X-radiation than normal tissue.

But normal tissue is always harmed by the process, only to a lesser degree. The treatment is given daily for five to eight weeks.

"External beam. There's some new data coming out of Seattle," he said.

"With implants."

"Yes, a combination of radiation therapy, and they're doing seeds plus external."

Seeds are permanently implanted pellets of radiation. They are inserted directly into the prostate gland.

"And for well differentiated, they've got about 94% disease-free at seven years," he said.

Well differentiated means that the cancer cells are similar in appearance to one another, and that they are similar to normal cells. Poorly differentiated means that there is a marked variation in the cancer cells. Like he'd said, you don't want a poor in anything.

"If you start looking at ten-year survival data for surgery in a low-volume disease, it's going to be around 97%."

"That's even better," I said.

"For low-volume disease which you have. You have a low-volume moderately differentiated tumor."

"Yes."

"I can't give you an exact figure. I can give you a ball park figure which is around 74%.

"74% of what?" Saralee asked.

I looked at Saralee. This urologist was totally confusing. We were being bounced about by statistics, some admittedly outdated or irrelevant.

"Of survival at seven years, disease-free."

"Is that with surgery or external?" she asked.

"With a combination," he answered.

"External beam radiation plus seeds," I said.

"Yes sir, external plus seeds."

"What would external only be?"

"Depending on who you read, around 68%. You can get a lot more radiation in with the two together. With some old data, there's five-year disease-free survival, again all stage B. And this is retrospective."

A retrospective study takes past treatment and compares that with the present population of patients.

"Is this the stage that Bob's at? Stage B." Saralee said.

"No, he's better than that. He's a stage A. Or increased PSA or T1c or whatever you want to call it. Whatever numbers I'm giving you are going to be better than that."

I thought, why isn't he giving me my numbers? I only cared about my own numbers.

"Because of my PSA?" I asked.

"Because of your PSA only. This is a retrospective study and was done by Paulson and a guy named Scardino, who is at Baylor. They took the patients from Duke and Baylor and lumped them all together, and they compared surgery, external beam, seeds, and a combination."

"What did they find?"

"With surgery, approximately 85% to 88% disease-free at five years. That's all stage B. That's a mirror image of what's confined to the prostate gland."

"Um hmm."

"External beam was no better than 65% to 68%. Seeds were no better than 58%. And the combination back then was no better than 58%."

I thought, why was he talking about "back then"? When would he talk about "now"?

"This data is old and retrospective, but it was the best that was done until the guys from Seattle got their data out. That's the best data."

"I've read a paper written by a group in Seattle," I said.

"What I do is to apply common sense to the best data out there. If the patient expects to live another eight or ten years or longer, has a good family history, and no health, breathing, or heart problems that would put him at risk for surgery, then I lean toward surgery."

"Okay."

"If he's going to live eight or ten years, and he's got some health problems that will make doing surgery a risk, then I lean toward radiation therapy."

"Uh huh."

"If the guy's not going to live eight or ten years, I don't do anything."

I began feeling gloomy, helpless, hopeless. I had so much to learn, and my life rested on my decision.

"You see what I'm saying? If you take all stage B cancers and you follow them for five years, only 45% are going to spread."

"Yes."

"55% are not going to spread. The problem we have is which ones are going to spread and which ones aren't. It remains a coin flip."

"Okay," I said, but I resented having my chances for life reduced to a coin flip.

"We also know a couple of things about why you don't need any fancy tests."

"But mentally I do need the tests."

"I know."

"If it were your husband . . . " Saralee said.

"I sent my brother to surgery without any X-rays."

Saralee laughed in disbelief.

"I love my brother dearly, but I sent him to surgery without X-rays anyhow."

"But I'm emotional," I said, tensely.

"I understand. Believe me, I understand."

"Okay."

"No problem. Percent positive bone scans."

A bone scan involves an injection of radioactive material that goes to bone and shows if the cancer has spread to bones. The urologist began drawing a graph to compare positive bone scans in relation to PSA levels.

"PSA levels, 10, 20, 60-plus. The positive bone scans are 0% from 10 and below and slowly rise, and you're way back here at 3.7."

He pointed to a spot on his graph, a low spot.

"Right," I said. "Exactly."

"Okay."

"I think there's a blood test to . . . " Saralee said.

"Right," I told her. "That's what he's saying. Acid phosphatase."

"Bob had an acid phosphatase done," she said. "The cancer had not spread to the bone."

"You can get fancy about that too, but again if they found that occasional cancer cell in your marrow, it doesn't mean that you have metastatic prostate cancer."

"Right."

"That test is kind of a moot point. Percent positive CT scan, PSA 25, 50."

He was drawing another graph.

"This a CT scan of what?" Saralee asked.

"Pelvis."

"Okay," she said.

"0% positive bone scan at PSA 25. And the flip side is if you do a CT scan, and you see a little 1 centimeter lymph node, you don't deny surgery to a young man because of the CT finding."

"Yes."

"Conversely, if you don't see a lymph node there, it does not mean you don't have something metastatic. It's a coin flip."

I thought, he'd do surgery for either one.

"I see CT scans on guys who come in here with a Gleason 8, 9, 10 and a PSA of 25 or 35. They can have CT scans if they want. But I'm going to save them with surgery."

"Do you use CT more than MRI?" I asked.

"I'm just looking for lymph nodes."

"I see."

"I'm just trying to find if it's in or out of the prostate gland. I'll do an intra-rectal MRI.

"I'm scheduled for that tomorrow."

"And I can tell which urologists know what's what by the tests they've ordered. If I see referrals from these small-town guys, the patient will come in with chest X-ray, bone scan, CT scan, MRI. The works."

"I'll probably want most of those done."

"They think they've got to do all these tests. You know, the patient doesn't need it. But it makes the patient feel better."

"Yes. I know you're not finished yet, but we'll have some questions later."

"If you don't, I'll be disappointed. All treatment options. Four we've already covered. Surgery, external beam, seeds, and a combination of radiation therapy with seeds. Cryotherapy."

Cryotherapy is cryosurgery. Doctors freeze the tumor with small coils filled with liquid nitrogen. These are inserted into the prostate under anesthesia. It is assumed that the cancer will be frozen to death.

"I talked with a radiotherapist who said, 'Don't even consider that.'"

"Don't even consider it. It's experimental and with a high complication rate."

"Right."

"There's watch and wait."

"I can't handle that. I need to deal with this pronto."

"Or hormonal therapy, not for you. You can put your cancer into remission with hormones. You can't cure it with hormones. There's a thing called hormonal down-staging."

"That's what Saralee's cousin was talking about. To shrink the gland before radiation therapy?"

"Yes. Then you follow it with surgery or . . . "

"Radiation. What do you think about that?"

"The numbers look really good. It may not affect the overall survival, but it will affect the drop in PSA profoundly," he said. Personally, I think it's a pretty good idea."

"What about liver toxicity?" I asked.

Liver toxicity can result from the use of medicines which are poisonous to the liver.

"Virtually none," he said.

"You're going to have three months of hot flashes, like a woman going through menopause."

"Uck," Saralee said. "You'll hate hot flashes. I did."

"And loss of libido."

"Double uck," she said.

"Okay, then let's look at time. Cancer starts out small. Two to four abnormal cells. Then it doubles."

"Uh huh."

"Cancer doubles for quite a while until it does one of two things. It raises your PSA, or it's palpable with my finger. So you had the cancer for quite a while, before it made your PSA go from 2 to 3."

"Right."

"So the growth curve is very flat, very flat, very flat. But all of a sudden, boom, you're in trouble."

"Yes."

"You're way down this growth curve," he said. "In other words, your internist found it as quick as it has ever been found."

"Actually, you found it, " Bob said to his doctor, "and I give you the credit for that."

"Your internist gets most of the credit, or whoever ordered the PSA."

"I ordered the PSA," Bob said.

"This is what I call a window of curability. Where the cancer is big enough to diagnose, but not so big that you can't cure it."

"How long is that window of curability?" I asked.

"It's anywhere from six months to two or three years, depending on how slow growing the cancer is."

"Yes."

"You've got plenty of time to seek second and third opinions."

"That's what I plan to do," I said.

"Yes, go. Definitely go. Don't worry about anybody. Seek all the opinions you want."

"Yes."

"The complications and side effects are roughly the same involving surgery or radiation."

"Wait a minute," Bob said. "I've heard that impotence is way higher with surgery."

"It's the same. I'll show you why."

He began drawing a picture of the location of the prostate gland.

"Your penis is here. Your sphincter is here. This is your prostate gland. Your pubic bone is here. Seminal vesicles will drain into here. Your rectum runs here. Your neurovascular bundles run out of your sacral plexus. Onto your prostate gland and out. Okay?"

"Yes."

I knew that Saralee had no idea of what seminal vesicles or neurovascular bundles or sacral plexus meant. I could explain all that to her later. Right now, I needed to deal with the facts.

"So if you cut it, and you look at it end on, when you're less than forty and have a nice little bitsy prostate gland with a hole in the middle of it."

"Right."

"Then you can take a cystoscope."

A cystoscope is a scope used to look into the bladder.

"And you can look straight in, and it's wide open," he said. "The transition zone is here and here."

He pointed to either side of the prostate gland he had drawn.

"Older than forty, it enlarges, and you end up with a much larger prostate gland."

"Uh huh."

"The part you're born with gets pushed to the back, and they call that the peripheral zone. That's where 90% of all cancers are."

The doctor pointed to his drawing.

"The rectum is sitting here, and the neurovascular bundles are sitting here."

The neurovascular bundles are cord-like structures that run down both sides of the prostate near the rectum. The bundles contain microscopic nerves essential for erection.

The neurovascular bundles also contain veins and arteries that help surgeons identify their location. In the past, they were frequently injured during surgery, because doctors didn't know they existed or understand their function.

"If you do external beam radiation, 40% to 45% are going to be impotent, because you're going to burn the nerve."

External beam radiation is a form of X-ray directed to a specific area of the body to kill cancer cells. To a lesser extent, it also harms normal cells. It can damage the neurovascular bundles, which the urologist referred to as the nerve.

"If you use combination radiotherapy, external beam and seeds, You get in more radiation. Instead of getting 6,000 rads, you get 12,000 rads."

A rad is a standard measurement of radiation.

"All right."

"The safest way to maintain your potency is to take seeds only, but the problem you have is that you're not curing the cancer."

"The seeds only will not cure the cancer in my prostate?" I asked.

"Not as well."

How aggressively did I have to be treated to be well? To be cured?

"To cure the cancer with radiation, you're going to burn a nerve. And that's the problem," he said.

"Yes," I said, and thought, the nerve I need for an erection.

"When you do surgery, you try to peel out the prostate gland and leave the nerve alone."

"Okay."

"The older you are or if you are a heavy smoker or have diabetes, the worse impotence problem you'll have."

I had never smoked nor had diabetes.

"When you're talking about prostatectomy, are you talking about simple surgery or radical?" I asked.

"Simple surgery gets rid of part, but the peripheral zone is still there."

The peripheral zone is the edge of the gland where many cancers reside.

"Simple prostatectomy, you take your fingers . . . "

He gestured with his fingers as if they were the end of a spoon.

" . . . and you scoop all this out, but the capsule remains.'

The capsule envelops the gland at its edge.

"Are you saying lymph nodes, too?" I asked.

"You'll get the lymph nodes sampled while you're there. Should you worry about them? No."

"So that when you're saying surgery, you're saying radical local surgery."

"You're taking the prostate and the seminal vesicles out."

The two seminal vesicles sit on either side of the prostate gland.

They store fluid that is mixed with semen and results in a man's ejaculation during intercourse. Without them, a man can still have an orgasm.

"Yes."

"What you got is a bladder. I'm going to draw one side."

He drew again.

"Seminal vesicle, sphincter, you're taking this out right here. What you're left with is a bladder, and you rebuild the bladder neck as best you can."

"How long do you wear a catheter?"

A catheter is a tube inserted through the urethra into the bladder. A bag at the end collects urine.

He paused, then said, "Ah. Up to two weeks."

"That long?"

"Yes. A man has two sphincters to his bladder. He has an external sphincter. Every time you go to the bathroom and shut your water off, that's the external sphincter."

He continued to draw as he spoke.

"You have an internal sphincter which is at the bladder neck and prostate. By definition, you are going to disrupt your internal sphincter. I'll rebuild it a little, but it's not God given."

"Uh huh."

"When you take the catheter out, most people are going to leak for a while. Until they learn how to control their internal sphincter. The things you can do to speed that up are lots of walking and lots of Kegel exercises."

Kegel exercises are done when a man urinates. He tries to shut off his urinary stream by tightly contracting the muscles in his buttocks.

"A woman has only one sphincter in her bladder. You're going to try to shut your water off with one sphincter. A couple of thousand of these exercises."

"Go ahead."

"Significant incontinence is less than 3% with surgery, and you're going to have 1% to 3% with radiation."

"Who does the surgery?" Saralee asked.

"If you want the surgery done in Atlanta, it would probably be me or . . ."

He wrote another doctor's name on his pad.

"Do we get to keep all the information and graphs you're making?" Saralee asked.

"Definitely. I'm making them especially for you."

"Thank you," she said.

"If you want surgery by the guy who designed the operation, you go to Saint Louis and have Catalona do it."

"Okay," I said.

"You have a lot of choices," he said. "None of them are particularly bad. You just have to decide what you want. Do you want your risk up front or do you want it down the road?"

"The three things that we want to avoid," Saralee said, "are incontinence, impotence, and an even more volatile gut and rectum, which he already has."

She had written this short list of things to avoid before we met with him.

"She's right," I said. "I do have an active gut."

"You're going to have a 10% chance or better that you're going to have radiation damage, because the external beam will bathe your rectum, too."

"Right. Is that permanent or temporary?"

"Most of it is temporary. You only get a 1% or 2% chance of severe complication rate from radiation. You may want to talk with a radiation therapist, too."

"I plan to."

"The difference in choosing a surgeon is only numbers. The

average urologist in private practice does six to eight of these a year. It's not enough to stay good. Those of us who have done a fellowship do fifty, sixty, eighty a year. Catalona does four or five a week. I sent my brother to Catalona. My brother lives in Memphis. There's nobody in Memphis I'd have touch my brother."

"How long is someone laid up?"

"Six weeks."

"Six weeks!"

"You can go back to work in three or four weeks if you promise not to help with the procedures. If you promise to just sit there and read the films."

"You can't even . . . ."

"You can't lift or strain for six weeks. You can sit there and read the films. If you do much more, you'll get a hernia. I guarantee it."

A hernia is the protrusion of part of an organ through the wall of the body cavity containing it.

"Where is the incision made?"

"Belly button to pubic bone."

I shuddered.

"If you choose external beam only, it's roughly six weeks of radiation."

"Yes."

"If you do combination radiotherapy, they'll give you four weeks of external beam radiation. Then they'll boost it with seeds."

"Right."

"It's not that big a deal."

I thought, not if you don't have the cancer.

"How long will he have to stay in the hospital with your surgery?" Saralee asked.

"Twenty-three-hour admittance. Actually if you get to the hospital early enough in the morning, you'll be home in time for dinner that night. Most of my guys want to go home that day. The food is better."

"Is Catalona's complication rate less?" I asked.

"Probably about the same. He's got the best published numbers for potency in the world. The guy who invented the procedure is out of Baltimore. His name is Pat Walsh."

I thought, didn't he already say that Catalona invented the procedure?

"It's a numbers game. If you pick nothing but young healthy patients with small tumors, you'll look real pretty."

"What happens," I asked, "if the man is impotent?"

"It's no big deal."

It was certainly a big deal for me.

"Is there a sexual drive?" I asked.

"One in ten men walking around right now are impotent that have had nothing to do with any of this."

"The general public?"

"One in ten. If I ride by a bus stop and throw a rock, it would bounce off two guys who are impotent. Extremely common. All ages."

I was amazed.

"Heavy smokers have it worse. Diabetics have it worse. But a lot of young guys have a venous leak and are impotent for no particular reason."

A venous leak means that blood that should be making the penis firm is leaking back into the general blood system, because the veins don't clamp down to keep the blood in the penis.

"There are drugs to deal with this. As long as you have a nerve and a sensation, you can rebuild the erection. That's not a big deal."

"But with radiation, they destroy the nerve, don't they?"

"Well, they destroy the neurovascular bundle, but the nerve is still there."

That was a relief.

"You've got to really go hard to get the sensation out of there. I guarantee you that you're going to walk away with a sensation and a sense of orgasm."

"Good."

"You may not be able to maintain a full 100% erection. That still counts as impotence. But you can tighten that up real easily. It's rare to have to put in an implant."

"What's an implant?" Saralee asked.

"An implant is a penile prosthesis that goes into the penis to provide erectile ability."

You pump up your erection with a fluid reservoir.

"Does one get an orgasm with that?" I asked.

"It has nothing to do with orgasm. It just provides you with erectile ability. A lot of the guys come in, and you treat them for erectile impotence with drugs. Once the dose goes in, the erection lasts from forty-five to sixty minutes."

I whistled.

"Wow, who would need an erection for an hour!" Saralee giggled.

I knew full well she'd love to cope with my erection for an hour.

"So there is sex after impotence, after the destruction." I said.

"Even if you're impotent, you can restore sexual ability in the vast majority of cases. So, everyone is satisfied."

"Would that be pleasant for him?" Saralee asked.

"Yes," He said. "The nerve is there. The problem is not sensation. The problem is erectile ability. And you can rebuild erectile ability four different ways. You can put a pellet of Muse into your urethra. It stimulates blood flow into the area. The new system is Intracorporeal Trimex injections."

"What's that?" I asked.

"An injection that goes into one of the two corpora cavernosa, the spongy areas on either side of the urethra that fill with blood during an erection. They communicate and the drug stimulates blood flow to produce an erection."

"Is that dangerous?"

"No. Or you can use a little suction device that will create an erection, and have a rubber band hold the blood flow in."

That sounded primitive and uncomfortable.

"You can actually put an implant in, which is the very last choice I recommend."

I certainly hoped it would never come to that.

"There are a bunch of different options. The easiest is the Muse system. I'll give you a pamphlet on that."

"Okay."

"I'll give you the best non-medical article I've ever read. It came out of *Time* magazine."

"Because this concerns both of us," I said.

"We still have a lovely sex life," Saralee added.

"You're going to come out okay," he assured us. "You'll have sensation. You'll have a sense of orgasm."

"What about the incontinence of urine? Is that any different between radiation and surgery?" I asked.

"No. Roughly 3%. And that's the severest of the incontinence where you have to treat it."

"Hopefully not."

"If you pick up a tennis racket or a number one wood and swing it hard, you'll have a couple of drops hit your pants. Because you don't have an internal sphincter. Same deal if you go to the Alpha tennis matches. Half those women are going to be wearing a pad."

I laughed.

"They've had two or three kids, and their bladders have dropped a little bit. The vast majority will have stress incontinence from exercise."

So would I if I opted for surgery.

"Are you sure of that?" Saralee said. "I'm almost sixty years old. I exercise a lot, and I don't have any stress incontinence."

"Join a tennis club and talk to the ladies in the dressing room. It's not do they leak. It's how bad."

"My friends don't complain about leaking," Saralee said. "That's hard to believe."

"So you lucked out. Have you had children?"

"Sure, two of them," Saralee said.

"Childbirth kind of weakens things. Time and gravity do the rest."

Saralee looked skeptical.

"As people get into their fifties and sixties, their bladder drops and they find themselves having trouble emptying, having recurrent infections, and having stress incontinence."

"I've had bladder infections," Saralee said.

"Yes?" he said, interested.

"I have lupus and before it was diagnosed, I had tons of infections. One after another. Anyway, we're here to talk about Bob, not me."

"You've been very encouraging," I told him. "I'm all mixed up as to what therapy to have."

"Don't worry about it."

"I called a radiation therapist that I know. He said, 'You must have radiation therapy. And then seeds after the external beam.'"

"That's one option."

"And you favor surgery. Does everyone favor his own specialty?"

"Yes and no. If you were about six years older, I'd push you toward radiation. If you were unhealthy, I'd push you toward radiation."

"He's very healthy," Saralee said.

"I'm so damn healthy. This has really hit me."

"Seven to ten years down the road," he said, "you have a decent chance of cancer showing up after radiation therapy."

That scared me.

"For a low-volume cancer, you have a 97% cure rate."

"With surgery."

"Yes. There's no radiotherapist that's going to promise you 97% at ten years. So, if you live ten years, you've got a decent chance you're going to break your radiation."

That sounded awful.

"The complication rate is no different. You drop 12,000 rads of radiation in there, your complications are roughly the same."

The urologist also told me of a local doctor to stay away from, who was famous enough to attract patients from other cities.

"He's a good marketer," my urologist said.

"Okay. Thank you."

I was grateful that he would level with me and wouldn't let me fall into bad hands.

"Anybody that puts together a color brochure and mails it to patients, soliciting business, is not my kind of doctor."

"Nor mine."

Even though surgery seemed a hideous prospect, my urologist was an honorable man.

"Tell me about Emory," I said. "Are they well known?"

"The guys at Emory do a perineal prostatectomy, and there's a higher chance of impotence."

A perineal prostatectomy removes the prostate gland by entering through the perineum, that area of skin between a man's scrotum and his rectum.

"The chief of urology at Emory does a really good perineal prostatectomy."

"But higher . . . "

"Higher impotence."

"Is the cure rate the same?" I asked.

"Yes. Cure rate's the same. But if you come between the scrotum and rectum, you have to come to the nerve first."

I laughed anxiously. With nerve loss, I couldn't have an erection.

"I and the urologist whose name I've given you do the highest volume on this side of town. What you want is a volume player."

"Um hmm."

"It's the same deal when you fly to Europe. You want your airline pilot to go there fifty, sixty times a year rather than six or eight times a year."

"You and that other urologist, can you work together on me?"

"No. He's my best competitor."

"Okay."

"Where's he at?" Saralee asked.

He told her his address and the name of the hospital where he did surgery.

"We've read about that hospital. It has the largest prostate cancer department in the city," she said.

"They had an ad in the paper yesterday," I added.

"Yes, that's junk. That's all it is—marketing."

"Hmm."

"What they've got is maybe twenty urologists from around the city who operate there. One urologist per 45,000 people. It takes 45,000 people to support one urologist."

"Oh."

"You've got a couple of million patients who are all coming there. You've got all the bells and whistles. This is all marketing."

There was a knock on the door. The last nurse indicated she was leaving. The office was officially closed.

"What surgery would need six weeks for recovery?" Saralee asked, perplexed.

"Radical prostatectomy. As far as driving a car, three weeks. As far as going to work, two to four weeks. Depending on how you feel."

"All right."

"The catheter comes out in a week. You might not feel like working then."

"Do men wear a condom?" I asked.

"Men wear a diaper."

"A diaper," I said with revulsion.

"You see it all ways. Some people, you take the catheter out, like Schwarzkopf. He had his catheter out, he was dry, day one."

But we're not all exactly like Schwarzkopf, I thought.

"If you read the *Time* article I'm going to give you, he was dry. But he was exercising. If you're walking, with good pelvic muscles and good pelvic tone, you're going to get continent a lot faster than the computer nerd that sits and plays with the computer all day."

"We walk four miles in an hour, or we work out on a ski machine for twenty minutes every day," Saralee volunteered.

"You should be fine."

"Yes," I said and hoped it would work out that way.

"What happens is your catheter comes out, and you're incontinent. You're wearing a pad."

I thought, like a menstrual pad.

"Then, you'll be dry in bed asleep. You'll be dry when sitting quietly in a chair. When you leak is when you stand, when you strain to get up. That's stress incontinence."

Stress incontinence seemed to be involved anytime you moved.

"Then you'll be leaking when you're out working in the yard."

"I do no yard work. We live in an apartment."

"Or stooping and picking something up."

It sounded as if I'd be leaky forever. The eternal sink with a dysfunctional faucet.

"You'll slowly get better."

"How long is one in the hospital with the surgery?" Saralee asked.

"Three days, plus or minus half a day. That's pretty quick."

He had said earlier that I'd only need twenty-three hours of hospitalization. That I could start early and be home in time for dinner where the food would be better.

"You've got the basics."

"Right."

"You just need to go to all the doctors, and decide for yourself. Don't let anybody put on a white coat and say, 'This is what you've got to go do.' You've got to choose, because you're the one that's got to live with it."

"And that's why I get so emotional about deciding," I said.

I sounded like a raw kid and felt bowled over.

"The radiotherapist told me that radiation is what I have to do. Talking to you now, I think surgery is what I have to do. I bounce about."

"You shouldn't think . . . "

"And Saralee is much more cool-headed than me about this."

"Well, it's not my body, but it is my life," she said.

"I don't tell people what to do. I don't put on a white coat. And it's worked out real well for me."

"Good."

"Two-thirds of what I do is because a patient sends a friend or a relative or a church member or whatever. So if the patient's well and happy, he's going back to church and saying what a great guy I am."

"True."

"And I'm not dependent on physician referrals. This means I can go into the hospital, and, if someone makes me mad, I can tell him what I think of him."

"That's right."

"So if the patient's cured from cancer and happy, I don't care what he's chosen. As long as he's happy. I want you to make your decision."

"Yes."

"If you want surgery and are concerned about every opportunity to maintain full potency, then you need to go to Catalona."

"Hmm."

"Then you've got a decision of a combination of radiotherapy. It's not a problem. You can get it in Atlanta."

"Yes."

"You say I want the best numbers published in the world, then you've got to go to Seattle."

"Okay."

"And you don't have to worry about my ego, or anybody's ego. You say, 'What's better for me?' That's where you go. If anybody's going to let their ego get into it and say, 'You should have gone to me or Joe Schmo,' don't worry about it."

"Oh, I'm not worried about that."

I fully intended to use diligence and make up my own mind.

"All I am is a facilitator," he said.

"Well, I respect my internist for sending me to you to you for the ultrasound exam. I'm very pleased with what you did."

"Thank you."

"I like the aggressive way you biopsy."

"I do the best I can."

"You were trying to get all the areas. Thanks."

"My dad had prostate cancer, and my brother had it at fifty-two. I have a very good chance of getting it, too. It's been in my family history. I figure if I'm as user friendly as possible, maybe it'll smile on me when it comes. Because it's coming."

"Is that why you went into urology?" I asked.

He told us that his dad had been an old-time urologist who worked six twelve-hour days and half a day on Sunday. That soured him on urology, so he took a math and sociology degree. Then, he decided that he had to get a medical degree. He rotated on urology for one month and got hooked on the specialty.

"I was born to do it. The personality types were my personality types. The surgery was the kind that I liked doing."

"How so?"

"It had a high diagnostic accuracy, rather than the exploratory stuff general surgeons do. We know what we'll do before we get there. There's no guessing."

"That's what attracted me to radiology. Its diagnostic accuracy."

"How many radical prostatectomies do you do a year?" Saralee asked.

"I do probably two or three a month. It waxes and wanes. I do over fifty a year."

"What is the percentage of impotence with surgery?"

She meant to pin him down.

"50% to 70% potency retained with surgery."

"Okay, so it's . . . " I continued.

"Yes, 30% to 50% you're going to lose your erections with surgery."

There was a long pause while that sank in.

"We've told you. Sex is important. It's not as important as curing the cancer, but I'd love to have both."

Overwhelmed, I continued, "I can't think of any more. That was really thorough."

"I want you to know what's going on."

"I'm so confused. I don't know if we should even go to Italy in October."

"Do all your research. Get your plan made. Go to Italy. And if you want to take a urologist along, that would be fine, too."

Saralee laughed.

"Come back and have it done, so you can quit worrying about it."

"I hope I have enough time to make my mind up by then."

Today was September 3; I had a huge decision to make in exactly one month.

"Get your plan made before you go. Schedule what you want done."

"That sounds logical."

"Otherwise, your whole plane ride over and back, all you're going to be thinking and talking about is . . ."

"No," I interrupted him. "I'm making a promise that we're not bringing the subject up, once I've made my decision."

"Good."

"Bob will have to decide," Saralee said. "He's a physician. He has much more insight into medicine than I do."

"Yes, but right now, he needs to drop the physician role, take the white coat off and be a patient."

"Exactly," I responded. "I'm really at that point, Saralee. When I look at my MRI, I won't know what I'm seeing."

They don't do MRIs at my 29-bed hospital, and I've never learned to read them.

"It's not going to change anything. You need something done," he said.

"Yes, right."

"These tests are like taking aspirin. They make you feel better, don't they?"

"More or less. You know, I never had an insurance bill, until I got Medicare. Now I'm eight months into Medicare and bang."

"Yes."

"With an involvement of only 5% of the gland," Saralee said, "does the whole gland have to be removed?"

"It's all or none. It's a multi-focus disease. You'll find bits of cancer you didn't know were there."

"And you think the 30% to 50% of loss of erection with surgery or radio, radia, radiation can be reversed," Saralee stuttered.

"When I had hypertension, my internist put me on Zestril to lower my blood pressure. I don't know if the impotence happened because I was turning sixty-five or if it was caused by the medication. I have an intermittent problem with that now."

"We can fix the intermittent problem. You'll get an idea of what's coming. I'll give you a dose right now. You have a 3% chance that your erection won't go down."

Saralee giggled. I knew that giggle. It sounded like fun to her. The longer I'd stay erect, the better she'd like it.

"What can I do if my erection won't go down?"

"Go to a hospital emergency room. The doctor will give you an Epinephrine shot to let the blood flow out."

"That's also used for allergic reactions."

"Yes. If you're nervous about having it done at an emergency room, I'll give you the shot.

"The drug I'm going to show you is called Muse. You put a little pellet into the urethra, and it's absorbed into the erectile body. It increases the blood flow, and you get an erection."

"Um hmm."

"Or you can use Trimex. The Trimex injection is done with a little thirty-gauge needle."

"The pellet sounds like a much . . . "

"Yes, that's a much safer way, because you're not using a needle. And when you do Trimex, you can only do it ten, twelve times a month. Because you're actually violating the space with a needle."

"Okay. Ten or twelve times a month."

"With the Muse you can do it two times a day every day."

"Is that all?" I asked jokingly.

"Sorry."

Saralee laughed.

"So it's much safer," he said.

This guy really wanted to help me. I liked him. Did I like him enough to let him cut me open from my belly button to my pubic bone and gouge out my prostate from deep within its bony crater?

"You're well away from the nerves. You're not doing anything there."

"I see."

"I'd do this all day long."

"And it has no hormonal effect that could influence cancer of the prostate?" I asked.

"Not a bit."

"I see. That sounds great."

"Let's go get you a dose."

"How long will it take to take effect?" I asked, as I followed him from his office.

"Ten minutes. I'll rent you a room. Oh, heck, you're a doc. I'll let you take one home."

"Okay," I said, relieved.

I did not relish driving through rush-hour traffic with a hard-on. He gave me three white packets. Each one held a different dosage of Muse.

"Sounds like a fun evening," Saralee said.

We were both due for some fun. Overdue. When we left the urologist's office, it was so late that rush-hour traffic was abating. We were both exhausted.

So much information to absorb. And this was only my first consult.

I needed to key down. To stop playing doctor. Saralee had a quick cure for that.

"I think we'll share a bottle of decent champagne."

She pulled a bottle of Heidsieck Monople from the refrigerator.

Saralee had stocked our wine cellar with cases of that wine at close-out price. I wasn't worried we'd run out of it any time soon. What I was worried about was my time left to live. Best not to think about that now.

Saralee grabbed two champagne flutes and said, "Where do we drink this? Offices or bed?"

Offices refer to our two leather armchairs in the living room. We view downtown from there, and sunset would soon be reflected on the skyscrapers.

"Offices for a while, then bed," I said. "I'll be with you in a minute."

From my study, I called my internist and asked whom he preferred as a surgeon for me.

"That's hard to say. If you weren't pleased with the result, I wouldn't want to be responsible," he said.

Generally full of ideas, my internist's passive response seemed ominous. I needed to think this surgery thing through alone. I joined Saralee and drank champagne.

"When are you taking a sex cookie?"

Saralee likes to name things. She was referring to Muse.

"Very soon."

I took one. It worked.

SARALEE

The next morning Bob was scheduled for an MRI. We were fortunate to find a spot in the hospital's crowded parking lot. Someone was pulling out.

Inside, we were directed to an outpatient reception area, a huge and crowded room. We went to the desk, and Bob was given forms to fill out. We sat down together. The waiting room was furnished with an assortment of chairs almost as varied as the people who sat on them.

It's appearance was scruffy, as if it could use a thorough cleaning. The mass of people made me feel as if we were on a conveyor belt, part of a mechanical process, dehumanized.

We waited until a receptionist called Bob's name. She directed us to a smaller waiting room for outpatient radiology. Though not as crowded, that room looked equally dingy.

Eventually, we were led to a third waiting area. It had only two scuffed chairs with a table between them. Soon, a woman emerged from an adjacent room in a white examining gown. She parted two curtains beside us and went into a cubicle that served as a dressing room.

When she had finished dressing, a technician gave Bob a white dressing gown and told him to strip. He handed Bob a key for a tiny locker, where Bob could store his valuables and metal objects, such as his watch.

"We'll put all of our valuables into my purse and store that in the locker. I'm going with Bob into the MRI, " I said. "Okay?"

"Sure," he said.

"I don't want him to feel alone there."

"I understand. I'll put a chair in the examining room for you."

We walked into the room the woman had recently vacated. I got my first look at the Magnetic Resonant Imaging machine. It was a long white tube with a curved examining table protruding from one end. Bob lay down on the examining table.

A young doctor, alert and energetic, walked in and introduced himself. He looked about the age of our kids, in his thirties. Bob introduced himself, too, and they shook hands.

"What I have to do now is a little uncomfortable. I apologize in advance," he said.

"No problem," Bob said. "I've already had an ultrasound of the prostate. A rectal probe was inserted then."

The doctor positioned Bob on his side with his knees pulled up toward his chest. I got my first glimpse of the probe, covered with lubricant jelly to make it easier to insert.

The probe looked like an oversized penis with a tip the size of a tennis ball, only smooth and shaped like a glans. It was the world's biggest dildo.

"Please relax your anal sphincter as much as you can," he advised. "I'll be as quick and efficient as I can."

Bob was facing me as the probe was inserted. His anus faced the doctor. I could not see him insert the probe. Only Bob's pain.

Once the probe was in place, and a balloon was blown up in the rectum to hold the probe in place, Bob sat up and massaged his pelvis.

"Can you tolerate this?" the doctor asked.

"I think so," Bob said. "I just need a minute to become accustomed to it inside me."

He patted Bob on the shoulder and said, "I feel we know each other a great deal better now that we've gone through this together."

The doctor was affable and charming. He had a lovely bedside, or rather tableside, manner. He left, and the technician took over.

"I'm going to slide you into the capsule now," the technician said.

"For the first seven minutes, I need to position you with your arms stretched above your head."

He was slowly sliding Bob into the capsule.

"Have you ever had an MRI before?"

"No."

"I always tell first-timers to keep their eyes shut."

The experience of being shut up inside an MRI machine tends to be claustrophobic, as Bob's brother had warned.

"Okay. Say, is there any music that goes along with this?" Bob said.

The technician held up a pair of earphones and said, "There is, but you won't need them. You've got her."

He pointed at me.

"You can have ear plugs if you want," he said and handed me a pair.

"I won't need these. She'll be my music."

"Yes," I said. "I'll sing 'Funny Valentine'. It's my favorite love song."

"Swell," the technician said. "I'll be in the next room, and I'll call out the sequences to you."

He left. All I could see of Bob now were his outstretched arms. All the rest of him was hidden inside the capsule.

"First sequence, seven minutes," the technician called through the intercom.

A series of clanging and banging commenced that prohibited any singing whatsoever. The earphones wouldn't have obliterated that noise. It was a combination of the worst aspects of John Cage and Philip Glass. With the volume full blast.

We had anticipated the possibility of claustrophobia. We hadn't known about the sound effects. I reverberated with the din and sat as quietly as possible. I couldn't communicate with Bob inside the capsule because of the commotion. I hoped he was doing okay.

After a series of sequences and cacophony that seemed to last far longer than seven minutes, the technician came back into the examining room, slid Bob part way out of the capsule, and repositioned him with his hands at his sides.

"Honey, how are you doing?" I asked.

"Pretty well. The claustrophobia hasn't got me."

"Wonderful."

"The noise sure has."

"Me, too. 'Funny Valentine' will have to wait."

"I'm lucky I don't have arthritis. It would be darn hard for me to keep my arms stretched up that long with arthritis. I guess that's lucky."

"You're lucky in lots of ways."

"I'm lucky to have you."

"And I, you."

The sequences began again and with them the sound effects. Now I could see the top of Bob's head inside the MRI tube. For over forty years, he has played many roles in my life—friend, brother, lover, husband, benevolent father, and co-parent.

Looking at the top of Bob's balding head, I saw what appeared to be a fontanel. He was now my babe, too. I walked close to him inside the machine. I could have reached out and touched his fontanel. I could have stroked his bald spot. But I didn't dare.

He had that gizmo stuck way up in him. He was wrapped up in the MRI tube. The noise was atrocious. He didn't need me as another distraction.

I saw red lights on top of the machine, a timer that counted the length of each sequence backwards. I riveted my attention on the timer and wished the sequences away. Eventually, my wish came true.

The technician came back into the examining room. He slid Bob out of the tube and removed the probe. Bob was free to dress and leave. He dressed and went to a bathroom down the hall to clean off the lubricant.

I would learn later that an up-to-date MRI machine made less noise.

Bob told the technician that he wanted to meet with the radiologist who would be reading his MRI. We were told to sit in the radiology waiting room for ten minutes. This would give the radiologist time to evaluate the study without our peering over his back.

Then, we were led to the radiology reading room. Like the doctor who had inserted the rectal probe, the radiologist looked the age of our children. Bob's study was hanging on the illuminated viewing boxes.

The radiologist told us that, as far as he could tell, the tumor was self-contained. It had not spread beyond the prostate gland. He thought he could see the tumor low on the left side of the gland, below an area of hemorrhage that was residual from the biopsy. Basically, the cancer was confined to the prostate gland.

Bob hugged him.

He gave Bob a copy of the MRI series and promised to fax a formal report as soon as it was dictated and written. The report was on our fax machine the next day, two pages full of encouraging words.

"The prostate gland capsule," the report said, "is smooth without evidence of tumor invasion through the prostate capsule. The fat plane between the prostate and the rectum is intact. The seminal vesicles are normal . . . without evidence of tumor extension into the seminal vesicles."

The tumor seen was one centimeter in size, about a third of an inch. The visualized skeleton was intact and without visible evidence of metastasis.

I had settled into a uniform that I wore daily, a navy blue suit that didn't wrinkle or show stains. I thought of it as both protective armor and as a cocoon.

It was a sunny day, and we decided to leave our car parked in the lot at the hospital. We crossed the street and walked to our appointment with a radiotherapist. We passed medical office buildings and the hospital itself, until we reached a building at the bottom of the drive with a large sign.

The sign said Cancer Center.

The reality of that sign hit me like an explosion and an earthquake combined. The sun glared on the sign. My navy suit was neither protection nor cocoon.

Cancer Center. This couldn't be happening to us. It was impossible on such a brilliant day with my husband beside me and holding my hand. We had always been so blessed. We were being catapulted from paradise into hell.

I blinked my tears into my nostrils and swallowed them. Bob opened the door, and we walked into a new world called Cancer Center.

In an empty waiting room, Bob picked up the registration forms at the desk and filled them out. I watched an aquarium filled with rare fish, like the one in our dentist's reception room. Supposedly, the fish comfort and tranquilize the patients. That didn't work for me.

A man entered with a hole in his neck and a triangle of dark marks beneath it.

"What are those marks on his neck?" I whispered to Bob. "The ones just below the hole."

"Tatoos that mark the margins of his external beam radiation scope," Bob whispered back.

The man left the reception room for his treatment and, when he returned several minutes later, he left the building. We were alone until a receptionist led us back to a treatment room.

There was an examining table, a stool, and a chair. I sat on the chair. Bob sat on the stool. A water faucet leaked in the corner, a reminder of the perpetual leaky faucet of urinary incontinence.

"Why are we here?" I asked. "Doesn't he have an office?"

"I don't know," Bob said.

"Isn't this supposed to be a consultation? Not an examination?"

"I don't know."

I think Bob was equally anxious. We sat, silent as stones. I listened to the leaking faucet. Chinese water torture.

Eventually, the doctor joined us and sat on the examining table. His legs, hanging over the edge of the table, were crossed. He was incredibly casual and equally young.

I forgot to turn the recorder on. Where would I have put it anyhow? On the floor between us? Maybe on the examining table beside him.

The doctor told us things we already knew about surgery. It was a one shot treatment. You'd need a catheter for a few weeks afterwards. Surgery had better survival rates after seven to ten years.

If we choose external beam radiation only, Bob would have treatments for seven to eight weeks. There was no incontinence with external beam, but there was bladder and rectal irritation.

We learned that you can have radiation following surgery, but that surgery is more difficult after radiation. The tissues inside that area of your body would have become scarred and very delicate for surgical procedures.

So, if we chose external beam radiation and Bob needed surgery later in his pelvic region for reasons cancerous or noncancerous, surgery would be difficult. The area would be friable, crumbly.

The radiotherapist told us about seeding which placed radiation in pellet form directly into the prostate gland. Using a rectal ultrasound probe for guidance, permanent seeds, radioactive implants, were placed solely in the prostate gland.

Bob would spend only one day and night in the hospital. He would be catherized after surgery. The catheter would be removed the following morning. In a week or two, Bob would feel recovered.

A 40% to 50% chance of urinary irritation could last a few months. Occasionally, there would be bleeding from the rectum a year or two later.

The doctor said that both surgery and external beam radiation had a 30% to 40% rate of impotence. With seeding, the impotence rate could be as low as 15% or 20%. He favored seeding.

Bob asked him how many implants with seeds he had done.

He'd done twenty or thirty in the last year.

Since the procedure requires a radiotherapist using the rectal probe and a urologist placing the seeds, Bob asked who the urologist would be.

His reply was the urologist we had seen yesterday.

I looked at Bob with amazement. That urologist had been so thorough in explaining our options. If he had done all these implants, why hadn't he said so?

Later, Bob asked the urologist why he hadn't mentioned doing the implants. The urologist told Bob that he put the seeds wherever the radiotherapist wanted them. He considered himself merely a technician during implant surgery.

Bob asked what form of radiation would be in the pellets.

His reply was Palladium-103. Neither of us had heard of Palladium-103. We had read about Iodine-125.

After a more thorough education, we agreed on Palladium-103 as a good alternative method of treatment. The half-life for palladium is 17 days; for iodine, it's 60 days. Half life refers to the number of days required for half the radiation to dissipate. In 60 days, half of the iodine radiation is gone. In another 60 days, half of the remaining radiation is gone, and so on.

Iodine is generally used for slower-growing tumors. Palladium is used for more aggressive ones.

The radioactivity of palladium decays in six months, while it takes twelve months for iodine to become inactive. So the patient recovers more quickly with palladium. The inactive seeds remain in the prostate without causing any reactions.

We left the radiotherapist's office with a new possibility. That Bob could be seeded only. We left with the instinctive feeling that this physician was not the man to do it. He did not strike us as experienced enough, and palladium was something we knew nothing about.

BOB

I worked on Friday. If I got involved enough in reading plain films—chests, arms, legs, hips, and other bones, GI series—barium studies of the gastro-intestinal tract from the throat to the anus, CT scans, mammograms, and ultrasounds, I could forget about my cancer for four or five hours.

It didn't work. I was Pigpen from a Peanuts cartoon with a cancerous dust cloud over my head.

I wasn't telling anyone at my hospital that I had cancer. In a small town, bad news travels like fire through a dry forest. I vowed nobody there would learn that I had cancer.

I speeded home. I'm good at exceeding speed limits on the interstate, just short of being stopped by the police and ticketed. The route to and from my hospital has become exceedingly boring for me.

Sometimes, I listen to the radio or to tapes. Sometimes, I borrow book excerpts from an audio-video rental store or the library. Sometimes, I read a little while driving. Saralee yells if she catches me reading while I drive.

By contrast, Saralee is an overly cautious driver. Many days, she doesn't drive at all. I help run errands on Mondays and Thursdays, when I don't work, and during the weekends, too. I usually do our driving. Two large shopping centers sit a couple of blocks from our apartment. She can walk to them if she wants anything. She claims there's not much left she wants—except me.

I escaped the Friday traffic and settled into our apartment. Her delightful self, albeit frightened, Saralee poured me a glass of wine and put it on my desk's coaster while I opened the mail.

At Theater Emory on Saturday and Sunday afternoons, we'd attend events related to the month-long celebration of Renaissance drama at the Black Rose, a reconstructed Elizabethan theater. We are both members of the steering committee, the board; Saralee is president now. Her Master's degree from Emory in literature, primarily Renaissance literature, would make the presentations especially meaningful for her.

Before the theater, we'd see what I could learn about my cancer at the medical library. I was perplexed by what I read. The surgeons all wanted to operate. The radiotherapists wavered between external beam, seeding, or a combination of both.

With surgery, I could have external beam later, if that proved necessary. The surgery sounded awful. If I had external beam radiation, surgery might be impossible afterwards, because of the spongy tissue. If I had seeds only, no surrounding nodes would be sampled or treated. Seeds were a relatively new process and didn't have the track record of either surgery or external beam.

There were reams of medical information available, more than I could assimilate. I didn't know what to do.

SARALEE

The excerpts from Shakespeare's comedies delighted me. The Black Rose has the capacity to simulate day or night; it was lit for night.

"Why are we doing comedy at night?" I asked a member of the theater department.

"Because that's when we need it most."

I reflected on that truth; our troubles seemed magnified at night.

Before and after the theater, we went to the medical library, where Bob did research. He would xerox pertinent articles and bring them home to read. He tried to make me read them, too. Whole. That didn't work. I couldn't understand the technical terms.

So he'd underline the most important parts. If I didn't understand what he had underlined, he'd explain. It was a mini-education in hell, something I wished that I'd never had to confront.

On Sunday evening, I attended a meeting of the architectural control committee for our condominium. We plan to redecorate the public areas of our building. Now, I had no interest in that project. I sit on too many committees.

The president of our committee knew I had a problem, though she had no idea of its magnitude. I asked to resign.

She said, "No. You have good taste. I want you to sit on my Christmas-decorations committee, too."

"What does a Jew know about Christmas decorations?" I asked.

"Enough," she answered.

Then, it was finally Monday, the day when we'd see the

radiotherapist we'd known for years. I thought, please help us make a reasonable decision.

BOB

We drove to his office, a few miles away from where we had all galloped horses together years ago, when we were totally invincible. The building was called a cancer center, but we had become accustomed to that title. Saralee and I sat together, while I filled out the usual forms. Before I finished, the radiotherapist came into the reception room to greet us. He shook my hand and kissed Saralee.

"It's wonderful to see you both. I'm sorry it's under these circumstances."

He explained to us that he'd never charged physicians before, but that the vagaries of billing and government supervision made it mandatory for every patient to be billed now.

I told him I knew all about that. I had to bill everyone, too, even my radiology technicians and the nurses who worked with me. Anyhow, the combination of Blue Cross and Medicare would probably foot most of the bill.

He led us into his office and sat at his mahogany desk. Facing him, Saralee and I sat side by side in commodious armchairs. She asked if she could record our conversation. He agreed.

"Let me tell you how implants got started," he said. "Back at the beginning of the century, they started putting implants into the prostate. Because they knew it was successful with other malignancies."

"Um hmm," I responded.

"So it's not a new concept by any stretch of the imagination. But, back in the '50's and '60's, people tried putting gold seeds and different isotopes into different parts of the prostate gland."

Isotopes are radioactive elements that decay within varying time—from less than a second to many years.

"Some patients were cured that way, but the numbers were small. It was anecdotal, and the complication rate was pretty high."

Anecdotal means that individual cases were described. No survey of all the people treated this way was kept.

"At Sloan Kettering, a couple of hundred patients had Iodine-125 implants placed suprapubically."

Suprapubically refers to the area above the pubic bone in the front of the pelvis.

"I got into that at my hospital. A lot of the urologists wanted us to try it, so we tried it. I did a lot of patients. I think I put seeds into a hundred or so. But the problem was getting an even distribution of the isotope, because it was done free-hand."

"Free-hand seeding would be uneven and risky."

"I have patients still around that I treated in the '70's, and they don't have cancer anywhere. But they're just a handful. We had a lot of patients who had complications. Mainly rectal complications, because we were getting higher doses posterially."

The posterior or back of the prostate gland is where most of the cancer resides. The gland backs up against the rectum there.

"So, I quit doing it. I said, 'No, I'm just not doing this any more. It has too many complications.' People reported in the literature that the complication rate was high. I abandoned it."

"Yes."

"Then, about the mid '80's, John Blasko, out in Seattle, started doing implants, but he went through the perineum using a template."

The perineum is the area between a man's scrotum and his rectum. A template is a metal grid with holes in it. The holes are evenly arranged horizontally and vertically.

"He'd space the needle holes at one centimeter intervals, and that's pretty damn rigid. I mean it's hard not to have an even spacing of the needles as you go through the perineum. It's that grid system."

"Right."

"What they were doing is using an ultrasound probe. Once they had ultrasound to visualize the gland, then they had a system in place where they could put a needle in."

"Yes."

"They knew where it was in the gland, and they could space it through the template. In stage T1's, a through c, that had a low Gleason and a low PSA."

"What's considered a low Gleason?" Saralee asked.

"I think at that time John Blasko was using 4 or 5 as his cut-off."

"Oh."

"These patients were treated with implants only. Five years later, 93% of them had no disease of the prostate gland. I think around 80% of them were biopsied again, and they were disease-free. Their PSA's remained normal, too. But you have to understand that those were highly selected patients."

"Right."

"And again, it's not randomized by any means. But it's hard to argue with 93%," Tom said and laughed, "at five years against anything."

"Even surgery?" I asked.

"Yes. Well, you'd probably do just as well with surgery. Absolutely."

"Oh."

"Bob, you've got to be careful about comparing radiation-treated patients to surgically-treated patients."

"As a general rule the radiation patients have more advanced cancer," I said.

"That's right. At least 50% of the time, the radiology patients have a higher range than the surgery patients."

"Yes."

"The way we know this is, if you look at just the surgical

patients, their preoperative clinical stage is upgraded 50% of the time. When operated on, they find capsular involvement or nodes or whatever."

"Oh."

"If you take the clinical stage, just what you can determine with finger and X-rays, and compare that to the stage after the surgery when you've got the prostate under the microscope, half the time the stage is upgraded."

That means more cancer is found when the gland is examined with a microscope than was initially suspected.

"They just published a new series of multi-hospital, multi-university groups of about 600 patients, and they found the same thing. If you just look at the surgery patients, their clinical stage is lower than their pathology stage, Bob."

"About 50%," I said and fretted.

"Does that mean that after surgery they're going to find he has more cancer than they suspected?" Saralee asked.

"Half the time. If you took 100 patients, 50 of them would have higher-stage disease than you thought."

"So do they automatically do radiation afterward?" I asked, frightened that I'd have cancer left even after the dreaded surgery.

"During surgery, they go in and take out lymph nodes."

Lymph nodes can easily become cancerous when you have prostate cancer.

"They're frozen."

At surgery, the pathologist does an immediate microscopic study of the frozen lymph nodes.

"If there's cancer in the lymph nodes, they close the patient up and he goes home. They send the patient to me for external beam radiation."

"I see."

The surgery was no sure cure either.

"Let's say they operate and the margins aren't clear," I said, "and they don't know that until after the surgery . . . "

"Yes?"

"Then what's done?"

"Then I think they should be radiated."

Surgery and external beam radiation. A double nightmare.

"Some urologists say it doesn't matter," he said, "but there are reports coming out to show that it does matter."

"I see."

"Earlier this decade, the positive-margin rate at my hospital in one year was 75%."

The positive-margin rate indicates cancer present at the edge of removed tissue.

"That's really high," I said and felt miserable.

"Do you know why? Because the poor surgeon is trying not to make you incontinent. Especially when he gets near the apex of the gland, he's very reluctant to really take a margin. And you get a positive margin right there."

"I see."

"To me, that means you have cancer remaining. I think to most people that's what that would mean."

"Yes. When you gave Blasko's 93% five-year survival rate with implants, does that mean survival or disease-free?"

"You can look at it any way you want. Survival, disease-free survival, biopsy-proven disease-free survival, PSA disease-free. There are a lot of ways to look at it."

"Right. With the numbers you gave me, I think it was 85% to 90% survival with external plus seeds."

"Right."

"Was that with the tumor confined to the gland?"

"Right. You have a relatively low Gleason. I prefer it to be even lower than it is if we're going with this approach."

"Yes."

"Did you read Partin?"

"I may have, but I don't remember."

"You can take someone's PSA, Gleason, and clinical stage and then predict what the probability of having nodal disease is. For a Gleason 6, PSA 3.7, clinical stage T1c, the probability is pretty low that you have nodal disease."

Nodal disease occurs when prostate cancer has spread to the lymph nodes nearby.

"Right," I said with a sigh of relief.

"If I were going to treat you, I would just treat the gland and assume you don't have lymph nodes involved."

"So you're saying, 'Just use implants.'"

"No. I would use the external beam to cover the gland and a little bit of surrounding tissue and then do the implants."

"I see."

"You have a small-percentage risk of having nodal disease."

"Right. Then why not routinely use pelvic ports?"

Pelvic ports are tattoo outlines that define a large area of the pelvic region. External beam radiation is aimed within those ports.

"Because the complication rate is too high. If you treat large areas with radiation, you're just asking for trouble."

"What sort of trouble?" Saralee asked, quiet but concerned.

"Well, he can have chronic rectal ulceration."

That means a continual ulcer in the rectum.

"A shrunken bladder. In some cases, it's necessary to treat larger areas. I personally don't think that 4,500 rads of external beam radiation is going to eradicate disease of the lymph nodes."

"I see."

"I can't go any higher than that."

"So that one doesn't kill microscopic metastases with 4,000 or 4,500."

"Theoretically, you can. Maybe there's a small group of patients in there, 1% or 2%, where that might work."

"Oh."

"But overall, if you have nodal disease, and this has also been shown in the surgical literature, the chance of developing distal metastases is so high that most of us wonder. If there's that risk, if it's that significant, you're not going to change the outcome for this patient."

Distal metastases means a far-ranging spread of cancer. A patient with distal metastases would be incurable with any treatment.

"There may be one little nodule of tumor that hasn't gone anywhere else in one particular patient, but I don't know how you'd find that patient."

"When people talk about external radiation now, do they talk about only the region of the prostate?"

"Right. It's called conformal radiation."

"That's what I was wondering. Whether you do that."

"Yes, I do. It conforms to your gland. We get a planning CT scan that cuts through the gland."

CT scans give cross-section views, slices of the gland.

"We use three-dimensional treatment planning and confine it to the volume of the gland and a little surrounding tissue."

"Does that include the seminal vesicles?"

They store the fluid that, mixed with semen, is emitted during a man's orgasm. Their fluid increases the volume of the ejaculation. A man can have an orgasm without seminal vesicles.

"I wouldn't on you. It would be extremely unusual for you to have seminal-vesicle disease from what we see on the MRI."

"Excellent."

"A reason we get MRI's is to see the seminal vesicles. The accuracy there is probably 85%, maybe 90%."

"Okay."

"I will try to keep your volume of treatment to a minimum."

"Would the volume be larger than the area removed at surgery?"

"Yes. A little bit."

"So you're getting more of it."

"Right. Probably a centimeter margin where they're not going to take a centimeter off the whole, top to bottom to sides of the periphery. They can't do that."

"I see."

"Especially posteriorly. They can't get a centimeter margin or they'd be in the rectum."

"Right," I said but wondered if I'd wind up with a permanently ulcerated rectum from external beam radiation.

"Bob's urologist mentioned that, during surgery, he'd be removing some part of the urethra," Saralee said. "That would cause one kind of incontinence."

"Right," he told her.

"Bob could relieve the incontinence with pelvic exercises," she continued.

"Right. But even with that, if Bob coughs or sneezes, he's going to leak urine."

"Oh," she said.

"That's the reason I decided a long time ago that I would never have a radical prostatectomy. Because I don't want to be incontinent for the rest of my life."

"Yes," I said.

"I think the risk of having some degree of incontinence is too high."

"A friend said that she knew a man who had surgery and found the residual incontinence maddening," she told him.

Saralee seemed comfortable talking to him. As friends, the three of us went back decades. He seemed equally well informed and capable as a professional.

"I think the risk of residual incontinence is on the border of 50%," he said.

"But there are degrees of incontinence," I said.

"Right. But some degree of incontinence is at 50%. The risk of total incontinence in Atlanta is probably somewhere around 5%."

"I see."

"Walsh claims he has about a 1% or 2%, but that's him," he said and chuckled amiably.

"I have three concerns," Saralee said. "First of all, Bob has a fairly volatile gastro-intestinal tract as it is. Incontinence is certainly another problem. And impotence is the third."

"Right." He paused then continued, "Now, I don't know how, on a practical basis, you can strip out the pudental nerve on either side of the prostate that sits in a groove in the gland. I don't know how you can strip that out and still do a cancer operation where you take a margin of tissue beyond the gland and leave someone potent."

The pudental nerve is in the neurovascular bundle. It's the nerve you want to save, so a man can still have an erection after treatment.

There was a long pause, while both Saralee and I pondered that.

"I just don't know how you do it," my doctor continued. "You know that nerve-sparing prostatectomy?"

"Yes," I said.

"Now that's what they're talking about. They strip the nerves away from the gland which bothers the heck out of me. I haven't seen your pathology report, but a lot of pathology reports say that perineural invasion is seen."

Perineural means around the nerve.

"My report didn't say anything about perineural invasion. It said one small portion of the gland showed undifferentiated carcinoma."

"Yes. Prostate cancer can spread along the lymphatics, the surrounding nerve fibers called perineural lymphatics. To strip nerves off right next to a cancer, hey, you're flirting with disaster. They want to save function, but I think you're taking a risk when you do that."

We sat silently and let that idea sink in. Thorough surgery implied impotence.

"Now that area is given a cancerocidal dose with radiation," I said.

"Same dose. Thereby, you may be impotent from the radiation."

"Yes," I said glumly.

"About half the time, the people are impotent. But of those patients who become impotent, if you look really closely at them, a lot of them were borderline impotent. They would have sex once or twice a year."

"Yes. Can this type of impotence be treated chemically?"

"If the nerve supply is still intact."

"See, with all this worry, I've had some of this impotence. The urologist gave me Muse pellets to put in my urethra. They are effective."

"Good!" he said and smiled encouragingly at me.

"Are you indicating that sometimes Muse doesn't work?"

"Yes."

"Oh, really," I said, as another worry sprouted.

"After the therapy?" Saralee asked.

"No, just anytime."

"It works."

"Good. We also have intracorporeal injections. They work."

Trimex is used for intracorporeal injections into the blood-rich areas of the penis, the corpora.

"Now Bob, several urologists have told me that next year they're coming out with an oral medication that will induce an erection."

We all laughed, and Saralee said, "Those will really be sex cookies."

"It sure ought to sell," I said.

"Yes," Tom chuckled, "a friend of mine says that he's testing it on patients."

"Oh."

"So there must be something to it. I don't know," he said and chuckled again.

"The doctor with the new pill sounds like a great idea," Saralee said.

"Yes," he said and paused. "There are also implants, and they have different kinds of implants. With one, your penis would stay semi-erect all the time, but it's erect enough for penetration."

"That sounds very uncomfortable," Saralee said.

"If not embarrassing," he said.

Saralee and the radiotherapist both laughed at the image of a man going around with half a hard-on visible. I found it unamusing. That man could turn out to be me.

"The other kind, that I really think is neat, is the kind where they put these two hollow tubes in the corpora."

The corpora are spongy chambers in the penis that become engorged with blood during an erection.

"And you have a reservoir system in the scrotum that you squeeze, and it inflates with fluid. You have a reservoir sitting somewhere in the pelvis that inflates those two things in the corpora, and you have an erection. So, afterwards, you hold the bulb and lose the erection."

I hoped that it would never come to that. I wanted to remain naturally manly, or, failing that, to use Muse or that new pill due on the market soon.

"Does one get an ejaculation with that?" I asked.

"Yes. Well, that brings up another point. I've had some patients tell me that they don't have an ejaculation. They have an orgasm, but nothing comes out."

"Oh," I said and wished we weren't considering this.

"After the treatment we're talking about," he said.

"After the radiation?" I asked nervously.

"We're not making babies, so we don't need sperms or ejaculations. As long as sex is something pleasurable for you and for me," Saralee said.

She reached her hand toward mine. I could tell she wanted to be consoling. Impotence and implants frightened her as badly as they did me.

"Obviously the main factor is survival," I said and stuttered on 'survival.'

"Right," Tom said. "I think the probability of getting rid of your malignancy is over 85%."

"With how many years of data?"

"Eight years. And they're supposed to come out with ten-year data any day now. I keep waiting for it, but . . . "

"In this one article that I read," I interrupted, "Blasko recommends either the seeds for local disease or external plus seeds for very bulky disease."

"He doesn't ever play with bulky disease."

"No? Not with external?"

"Or if you have anything over a T2a. The Gleason and the PSA are critical, Bob, in decision making."

"Yes," I said and thought, I have only a T1c.

"If you had a Gleason score of 4, I would recommend you have the seed implant, and that's it."

"That's what another radiotherapist we consulted with recommended," Saralee said. "Seed implant, period."

"With a Gleason 6?" he asked.

Well," I said, "what he told me was that since it's a 6, he'd recommend the palladium, not the I-125."

"I don't use palladium until you get above 7. And no one's ever shown that palladium has any superiority over Iodine-125, anyway. It's theoretical."

"Do you think I ought to have the pathologist review the slides and make sure that they're a Gleason 6?" I asked and hoped a pathologist might come up with a Gleason 4.

Then my radiotherapist friend would do only implants. I had confidence in him. So did Saralee.

"Yes. But they're usually pretty good at grading Gleason. They see so many biopsy slides."

"Can someone at your hospital review my slides?" I asked

"Ask them to send your slides over," Tom said. "I'll have our pathologists review them."

"Yes," I said, determined to shave a 6 down to a 4.

"Also, the MRI was not read by the radiologist you recommended," Saralee said. "He wasn't there that day."

"He saw it and called me. And he agreed with the reading."

"That was nice of him," I said. "We asked for him to review it."

My doctor laughed genially and said, "He did."

"Let's say you did the external beam, and I went to Blasko in Seattle for the seeds. Can you send sufficient information for Blasko to know what to do?"

Dr. John Blasko published a lot. His name appeared as the lead writer in several journal papers I had gathered from Emory's library. I was impressed by his findings.

There was a long pause while my doctor thought.

"Does he have to do his own CT and all those other studies?" I asked.

"He probably would."

"Oh."

"Here's what happens. You have the external beam radiation, and then, near the end of that, you have a volumetric study. That's an ultrasound, and they do polaroid images of the ultrasound screen. Starting at the base and going to the apex."

"Yes."

"My physicist takes those images and puts them serially into a computer. The physicist asks the computer to tell us where to put the needles so that we get an even distribution."

The needles he was talking about were actually thin tubes. Each tube would hold a number of radioactive seeds. The seeds would be released into the prostate, and the needle, removed.

"Now, I do not load the center. Because if you look at the dosimetry of an implant, it's hot anyway. Where Blasko had his complications was in the center, in patients who had previous TUR's."

Dosimetry is the amount of radiation dose and its placement in the gland.

TUR means transurethral resection of the prostate. It's the same thing as a TURP. It is used with men whose prostates have grown so large it is difficult for them to urinate. It does not require an incision. You go in through the urethra and chip away tiny pieces of the prostate and remove them through the urethra. This procedure eases bladder problems but puts the urethra through stress.

"Do you do even distribution or do you weigh more in the periphery?" I asked.

"I weigh it a little more in the periphery, but I don't implant right around the urethra."

"I see."

"And we don't have any side effects or complications."

"How many seeds are used?"

"That's higher than we ever used before. On average, it's about 85 or 90 seeds."

"How many cases have you done?"

"I've done probably about 150, something like that."

"Over what period of time?"

"Two years."

So he'd been doing about 75 a year, almost three times the number that the younger radiotherapist had done. But he had only a two-year track record with seeds.

"We're doing 5 next week."

"Would the external be done in this building?" I asked.

"You could do it here or at the hospital."

"How often would you come in and check everything?"

"Weekly."

"How do you keep the port exactly on the prostate gland?"

The port is the entrance area on the skin where a tattoo has been placed.

"We have a CT scan, a planning CT scan. That tells me right where your gland is. Remember I'm taking a margin beyond your gland."

"Yes."

"We're taking a straight AP."

An AP is an anterior posterior view, which means front to back.

"An orthogonal lateral, 90 degree film."

Orthogonal refers to a right-angle view from the AP which is a true lateral. With these two views, they'd be able to aim the external radiation directly at the prostate gland. At least it was accurate.

"We outline where I'm going to treat. And we take the CT and those films and put all that in the computer. And the computer tells us what the shape should look like."

"Yes."

"So we cut a block that fits your anatomy. And we make marks on your skin. Permanent marks. Little tattoos. Little dots."

"Uh huh."

"When you come in each day, they'll put you on the table. Right in the center of the table. They look at you, make sure you're as flat as you can get. They look at the lateral with a laser which should match that spot that's tattooed on your hip and should match the one suprapubic area."

"Good."

"So we've sort of triangulated it with lasers. And then, once a week, they take a film of those two fields, the front and the side."

"Yes."

"The way I do it is with a rotational technique. We know that point in space where the center of your gland is. And we set up those two bars and rotate around a point in space."

"I see."

"The beam is off over the bladder, and it's off over the rectum. So it's just coming in from the sides."

"I was reading that the prostate gland can change position according to the fullness of the bladder and the rectum."

"Right. It can, but that variation is small."

"I was thinking you'd probably have to urinate before each session."

"I think you could urinate before each one or don't urinate. As long as you do the same thing every time. But its not urine. It's feces that make the difference. That has been studied extensively. If you have a full rectum, it can push the prostate anterior."

"I see."

"Almost always, I include a little bit of pubic bone. If you look at prostates, they're really tucked in right under the pubis, and that's a bony structure. If you have a little pubis in your treatment field which is a centimeter margin, even if you had a full rectum and it pushed it, it can't go farther than the bone."

"Yes."

"So I'm not worried about anterior displacement. If you have an empty rectum, it could fall posteriorly. The maximum movement that anyone has ever been able to reproduce experimentally is only a centimeter and a half."

"Hmm."

"Bob, I'm just not worried about that. I don't think that happens on a daily basis. You may have a half centimeter at the most. It's probably more like a quarter of a centimeter."

"How many weeks of therapy will Bob get?" Saralee asked.

"Five weeks."

"Okay," I said. "The treatment itself takes only a minute or two, doesn't it?"

"Yes, about a minute. The set-up period is what takes up all the time."

"Is there a difference in the machines around town?" I asked. "Is one a better machine than another?"

"Better? I think the most important thing is good localization. That's what I call technique."

"I see."

"I think that's much more critical than the energy of the machine. Because the machine here is 6 MEV, and it does fine."

MEV refers to the strength of the voltage.

"So you have a 15 MEV machine. So what. You're still treating the same volume. You've got to worry about neutrons on the 15 MEV. You don't have to worry about neutrons on this," he said and laughed.

A 15 MEV machine produces neutrons which penetrate more deeply during treatment than does a 6 MEV machine. In using the 15 MEV machine, a potential risk is contamination of the treatment room.

"The total dose, the radiobiological dose, is exactly the same."

"I guess so."

"So I think technique is much more critical than the actual energy of the machine."

"You mentioned that Bob had an 85% chance of cure out to eight years," Saralee said in a frightened voice.

"Saralee, I can show you literature to support that," the radiotherapist said.

"What the urologist told us was that the survival with surgery and radiation are equal up to ten years," I said. "After ten years, the radiation survival, disease-free, goes down faster than with surgery."

"He's right. But he is talking about external beam only."

"Is external with seeds a different ball game?" Saralee said.

"Yes. The dose that I could give Bob using external and seeds is double what I could do with external alone."

He paused, then said, "At least double, if not higher. Which I think is going to translate into excellent local control."

"Good."

"If this cancer has already spread somewhere else, I don't care what you do. You can operate. You can do anything you want to. It's not going to work."

This thought made me feel miserable.

"So you have to talk about whether or not the cancer is controlled in the gland," he said.

"According to the MRI, it looks that way," I said.

"Yes. And if our assumption is correct that the disease is confined to the prostate gland, then you have to decide the best way to treat the gland itself."

"Are there any other options?" Saralee asked.

"There's nothing wrong with surgery. Don't misunderstand me. But the surgeons have problems."

"Right," I said.

"Their problems are that anatomically it's difficult to operate, because it's in a bony and confined space. It's a bloody operation. Exposure is very difficult. And because of those factors, I think they have a too high complication rate."

"Yes."

"It's not the surgeon's fault. The surgeon is a good technician, but it's just where the prostate is located."

"It's just where it's located," Saralee echoed.

"That's right. And if you're going to do a cancer operation, you're going to have some complications from it. Impotence and incontinence are the two big ones. Then there's a list of others that go along with the major surgical procedure."

"But, ignoring complications, are there studies going out a long enough time to say survival is different between the two, using the seeds?" I asked.

"We have data to support that."

"I see."

"An Atlanta radiotherapist has published a paper that's out to ten years. What he claims is that if you get a PSA after the procedure down in the 0.5 or below range, your chances are 95%."

"For how long?"

"Ten years."

"Is there any medical test that can determine lymph node involvement?" Saralee asked. "Something short of opening up the pelvis and scraping bits off of his lymph nodes?"

"No, what we look for is enlargement. Lymph nodes enlarge. You have to wonder why it's enlarged. In a setting where there's a malignancy in the area, you can assume that it's enlarged because of the malignancy."

"Yes," I said glumly.

"Now it may not be. It may be enlarged due to the fact that you've done a biopsy of the gland. Or you had an infection in the area, and that made the lymph nodes enlarged."

"Oh," I said more hopefully.

"But it's so crude. All you can say on the CT or the MRI is that there's an enlarged node sitting right there. Then you do a laperoscopic removal of that lymph node and see if it has cancer in it."

A laperoscopic removal involves a tiny incision. Much of the surgery is done with small scopes. So it is minimally invasive.

"In Bob's case there were no large lymph nodes, but it's only a presumptive diagnosis that he doesn't have a node."

"Right," I said anxiously.

"I think we have something now with radiation that's as equally effective as surgery, but it has fewer complications. That's why I advocate it."

"Do you think the survival is better, all things being equal, using external plus seed versus only seeds?" I asked.

"If you had a Gleason 4, I'd just do seeds."

"I see. Okay," I said and vowed I'd find some pathologist who would read my biopsy slides as Gleason 4.

"And you could probably just do seeds now and get away with it, but I would feel more comfortable . . . "

"Yes."

"I'm trying to put myself in your chair."

"Right. Right," I said and knew no one could understand how uncomfortable my chair was. "Well, I would feel easier with a nice margin."

"Right," Tom said sympathetically. "That's the difference. Yes, we can have it reviewed, and if the pathologist says, 'I really think this is a Gleason 4,' I'll do seeds only."

"Super."

"Do you understand what Gleason means?"

"It's the degree of differentiation."

Differentiation of cancer cells is shown by how the cells look under a microscope. Well-differentiated ones have distinct borders and clear centers. They grow slowly. Poorly differentiated cells are not so well defined and look cloudy. As the cancer grows, these poorly differentiated cells come together and form solid areas of malignancy.

"Well, they've seen more than one degree of differentiation in your tumor, and they've noted that."

"Right."

"What they look at is the predominant differentiation."

"I see."

"So they look at all the cancer, and they say 'Well, the predominant thing is a Gleason 4, over here, this one little area is a Gleason 8.'"

"So they average it all out."

"You have a primary and secondary differentiation. And you can have tertiary or quaternary differentiation. But the primary and secondary are the two numbers that you get. On the primary, 1 to 5, and on the secondary, 2 to 10."

"Yes."

"Okay. That's how they come up with the Gleason score. The predominant is one number. And the second most common degree of differentiation is the second number. They've noted on yours that there's one area of 4 differentiation. So, what I'd assume is that you have a 2 and a 4 or something like that."

What I needed was a 2 and a 2.

"They're noting that there's one little area that's maybe a little higher," he added.

"How can you get your pathology slides?" Saralee asked.

"I'll call the hospital where they're at and ask to have the slides sent to my radiotherapist's hospital for another evaluation," I told her.

"Okay. Ask them to send your slides over. That I would like to have them reviewed. I'm not telling you what he'll come back and read it as," my doctor said.

"Right."

"Well I'll tell you," I said, "it really is . . . "

"Tough," Tom said.

"Yes. It really is stressful."

"Yes," Tom said.

"I thought I was in perfect health."

Tom chuckled.

"And that nothing was ever going to go wrong with me."

Tom chuckled again.

"I work three mornings and early afternoons. Could treatment be later in the afternoon?"

"Sure. Just so it's the same time each day."

"When I got my radiology boards in '64," I said, " I was board certified in therapeutic radiology . . . "

My radiotherapist laughed.

" . . . nuclear medicine and diagnosis. What a joke."

He laughed louder and said, "it's a little different now."

"Oh, yes. That's why I say it."

"Well, I think they did away with the dual boards shortly thereafter," he said.

"Oh, yes. They had to," I said. "Radiology developed so fast you couldn't keep up with all three fields."

"1965 or '67. Something like that. If you decide to go this way, I'll show you our three-dimensional treatment plan. It's fantastic."

"Would you like to look at that now?" Saralee asked me.

"No," I answered her. "I don't need that now."

"As I see it, the external placement is less critical than the implants," I said to him.

"No. They're both equally critical."

"How much dose does the periphery of the prostate get with the implant?"

"Total?"

"No, with the implant only."

"You get around 12,000 rads with palladium and 16,000 with iodine."

"Wow. You can never get that in with external only."

"No."

"You only get about . . . "

"7,000 at the most. Some people are going to 8,000 now. I would be very fearful of going to 8,000 rads of external beam."

"Yes."

"Mainly because of the rectum."

"I understand."

"The implant dosimetry is really nice, Bob. We leave about half a centimeter of the posterior wall, the posterior-most row of seeds that we use. If you look at the dosimetry there, you're not getting a significant amount of radiation to the rectum."

"Well, I guess what I was concerned about is, if one of these seeds or two of them are off, will there still be enough radiation to knock out the tumor?"

"Yes. That's another good thing about having the external. Because going into the implant we know you've had an honest 4,500 centigrey already."

Centigrey is the universal measurement of radiation. It corresponds with rad.

"If one seed is off a little bit, it's not going to matter as much as if you had no external."

He turned to Saralee and said, "You understand that, don't you?"

"Uh, basically, I think so," she said.

"Okay."

"Externally you're going to give him 4,500," she said. "The 12,000 includes the external plus the implants."

"Well, it's probably going to get up to more like 16,500 total."

"That's really high," I said.

"Real good," he said. "You know, we've never been able to get that high before."

"That sounds good. I'll be safe then," I said but wondered about the complications of so much radiation.

"With ten years of experience, which should be coming up pretty soon, it may be that we'll look at cutting down on the amount. Maybe we'll cut back 2,000. Just to be safer."

"Um hmm," I said, even more worried about over-treatment.

"We may not need to go to 16,500. I don't know. Right now, we're not cutting back."

"Bob doesn't want to sit around with this cancer long before treating it," Saralee said.

"Right. Well, you know, when I used to treat Hodgkin's disease, everybody got 4,000."

Hodgkin's disease is a type of malignancy of the lymph nodes. If caught early enough, it can be cured.

"You had to be sure that you got 4,000. Now, we're cutting way back. To uninvolved areas we're thinking 3,000 or 2,500 is all you need."

"That's interesting"

"So things have changed over the years as to how we're treating them. But for right now, we're going to stick with this system. My brother-in-law has T1c with a Gleason 4, and we did an implant-only on him."

"Yes." I said and envied the lucky guy.

"We did it last year. He has not slowed down one bit. I mean, it has not bothered him in the least. His PSA is 0.2. They'll always be a little PSA, because you always have a little viable prostate."

"How the heck can it live with that high a dose? Is that potential for malignancy right there? The urologist's idea was to cut the sucker out."

Tom laughed.

"That way you know you can't have anything there," I said.

"That's fine. There's nothing wrong with doing that, and you know that. Bob, you might go through a radical and just breeze through it, but you've got to understand your risks. And in my opinion, the risks are too high."

"Well, let's say you have somebody fifty years old or forty-five."

"The recommendation would be exactly the same."

"No matter what age?"

"No matter what age. And, just for your information, I have treated men in their mid-seventies and low eighties with this same sort of regimen I'm talking about for you. They tolerate it beautifully."

"Yes."

"I tell these people that they probably don't need any treatment. The urologist tells them that, too. But they want something done. It's psychological."

"In general, are the malignancies more aggressive the younger the age?"

"Yes."

"Also," Saralee said, "the older you get, the worse your chance is of surviving surgery."

"Right," my doctor said. "Most urologists won't operate on you if you're over seventy."

"Dying is something else," I said and shuddered instinctively.

"How about that? I'm honest with these people. I tell a seventy-five-year-old guy, 'Look, you don't need any treatment.'"

"People who are seventy-five think they're going to live until they're ninety-five, I guess."

"And I guess some of them may. When do you cut off treatment? I don't know. But I can tell you this, with few exceptions, it's extremely well tolerated."

"I'm not worried about tolerating it. That doesn't bother me. It's survival . . ."

"No, but he is worried about tolerating the surgery," Saralee said.

"I'm not worried about tolerating anything," I said emphatically. "I want to survive. I have a will to live."

"Unfortunately, there is no clear cut advantage to either one," my doctor said.

"Do you find that men can continue working?"

"Yes."

"Even at the end of the external?"

"Yes. You may feel tired during the external. You may not. I've treated a lot of men who didn't feel tired. You may have some diarrhea. You may have some dysuria."

"What's dysuria?" Saralee asked.

"Burning when you urinate," Tom told her. "Bob, I have a guy right now who is a veterinarian and lives in Dahlonega."

Dahlonega is a town in the Georgia mountains about fifty miles north of where we were sitting.

"He rides a motorcycle in for his treatments," my doctor said and chuckled.

"Oh, brother," I said.

"He's about three or four weeks into treatment, and he's getting a little bit of burning right now."

"We'd planned a trip to Italy in early October as a fortieth-anniversary present. Should we cancel and start therapy immediately?"

"No."

"Okay. I'm exhausted. The stress is very tiring."

"I hope you guys have a great trip. Will you go to Venice? I love Venice," he said.

Saralee nodded.

"Drink a glass of *prosecco* there for me."

SARALEE

Alone on Tuesday, I worked out on my ski-machine, 400 calories burned away in twenty minutes. Then I sat down at my computer and tried to write.

Michele comes on Tuesday and cleans up our act. She's both a housekeeper and a buddy. She found me at my computer with tears running down my face.

"What's wrong?" she asked.

"Bob has prostate cancer, and I'm trying to write about it."

Michele put her hand on my shoulder. I stood up and hugged her.

"How bad is it?" she asked.

"Not bad at all. But he wants it taken care of fast. He's talking about surgery."

"What would that mean?"

"He'd be slit from his belly button to his pelvis. They'd gouge out his prostate gland and who knows what else."

"I'm sorry."

"He'd be out of commission for six weeks. Maybe even forever because of the complications."

"Like what?"

"I don't want to talk about that. I can't face it yet."

"Must he have surgery?"

"No, but I think that's what he wants."

"What other options does he have?"

"External beam radiation. He lies down on a table and they zap him with high doses of radiation."

"What does that do?"

"It burns the prostate and other areas surrounding it. Areas that he might miss having. Areas that I might miss his having."

"I see. Any other choices?"

"There's seeds."

"What are seeds?"

"Pellets of radiation put directly into the prostate. They give a much higher dose to the gland itself."

"Only the gland?"

"With seeds, yes. One doctor offered to treat him only with seeds."

"What does he think about that?"

"I don't think he'll buy that. Too short a track record with seeds alone."

"Oh."

"And neither of us thought much of the doctor who suggested it. Too young, too inexperienced."

"I can understand his wanting to go with a doctor he really believes in."

"There's watch and wait, too. He's definitely not going for that. Bob wants to be treated immediately."

"Saralee, with all these choices, the two of you will come up with something appropriate. You're both bright. He's a doctor."

"Yes, he's a doctor. But he's a patient now, too."

"When does he have to decide?"

"No time soon. But he's planning to decide before our trip."

Michele would feed Praise and play with him twice a day while we were gone.

"I think Bob and you will work this out. Go to the refrigerator. Pour yourself a big glass of wine. Drink it. Then try writing."

I followed her suggestion. I began writing and didn't stop until just before sunset. Then I enjoyed watching day turn into night. On this clear night, the lights from downtown skyscrapers gleamed.

Bob called as he does on Tuesday when we're apart. We frequently talk during the day, too, but his early evening call is our ritual. We talk about his day and mine. Mostly, we hug across the ninety miles of telephone line that separates us, say, "I miss you" a few times, and "I love you" more times.

He was going to Reynolds Plantation at Lake Oconee for dinner tonight. A country club with elegant homes surrounding the golf course and the lake. And delicious food; we'd eaten there frequently when we lived at the farm.

"What are the specials tonight?" I asked.

"Sautéed trout with almonds or pork tenderloin with shiitake mushrooms."

"Yum. Which will you have?"

"I haven't decided yet."

"They both sound like winners. Enjoy."

He didn't ask about my dinner. I diet on Tuesday. Later I munched carrot sticks and a handful of blueberries.

That evening I called Pat, the director at Theater Emory I coordinate with as president of the steering committee. I needed to tell her about Bob's cancer in case she wanted me to step down as president. I would have told Pat anyhow. She's a close friend whom I needed for support.

"I have no idea how my life and Bob's will work out in the near future," I said.

"Saralee, forget all about Theater Emory. Missy and I will take over until you sort things out."

Missy was my capable vice president.

"I have written an agenda for the meeting next week, but it's in long hand on a legal pad," I said.

"Good. Fax it to me."

"I don't know if you can read my chicken scrawl."

"Fax it to me anyhow. I'll take over from there."

When Bob and I arrived at the steering committee meeting the following Wednesday, Pat had prepared my agenda with enough copies for everyone present.

The phone rang as soon as I put it down. It was Mark, talking in his silkiest voice.

"I just want to know how everything is going," he said.

"It's going fine," I lied.

"May I speak with Bob?"

"He's not here. He sleeps in a motel near his hospital every Tuesday."

"He's doing all right?"

"Of course."

"Good. That's what I want to hear."

"This morning Bob did some radiology. This afternoon he played bridge with his regular Tuesday group. Now he's probably having dinner at Reynolds Plantation on the lake."

"It all sounds lovely," he purred.

"Lovely," I echoed. "Thank you so much for caring."

The tender care that our family and friends gave us mattered greatly. On Wednesday morning Ned came to visit me. His had been a long marriage like mine.

We sat together on a sofa in my living room. Bob and I had spent a week dodging workmen, while they installed marble floors in the living and dining rooms a few months ago.

"Your new floor looks great," Ned said. "It makes the rooms look enormous."

"Yes, and reflects the sky and clouds, too," I said. "May I hold your hand?"

"Sure."

He covered my hand with his large one.

"Ned, none of this is going to make any difference to me if Bob doesn't survive."

"None of what?"

"None of these trappings. None of my life. Without Bob, I'm a goner."

"That's not true. You have interests of your own. You have friends of your own."

"That wouldn't be enough to make me want to go on living."

"You're a writer. You're a docent at the museum. You're involved in the theater."

"I couldn't bear going to the theater alone."

"You'd invite a friend."

"That would be insufficient."

"You're not being reasonable. It seems you do most of the arranging for the two of you anyhow."

"The social arranging. Travel plans. Minor things like that."

"That's not so minor."

"Bob and I have been together most of my life. I couldn't bear living without him," I said and tried not to cry.

We sat quietly, until I regained some composure.

"Saralee, people do adjust. You'd have to give yourself a year."

"I wouldn't last a month."

"What do you mean?"

"That I would want to lie down in bed with some pills and a great bottle of Burgundy, fall asleep, and never wake up again."

"That's absurd."

"No it isn't. I can't even cook without Bob anymore."

"Why?"

"I'm tired of cooking after forty years of it. He pitches in and helps. When we make roast beef, he mashes the garlic and spreads it on the roast. Raw garlic makes my fingers smell for days afterwards."

"You could wear rubber gloves."

"And who would I make the roast for anyway?"

Ned had no answer for that.

"Ned, I care more for Bob than I do for myself. My center of focus is not myself."

"Really?"

"I'm dependent, needy. He's more than half our team."

"You'd find someone else to team up with."

"Nobody who'd matter. Nothing like what I've had. It's been a remarkable forty years. Not every day, but most of them."

"Yes."

"You take forty years of anything. Not all of it works."

"I agree."

"Most of ours has worked. If our life together ends . . ."

"Promise me you'd wait a year," he said.

"I'm making no promises."

I stood and said, "You've listened to enough of this. I need a hug before you go."

He gave me a fond hug.

I spent the rest of Wednesday writing and crying, sometimes both at once. About three, Bob arrived, and his vitality filled our quiet apartment. The phone started ringing. A fax arrived.

BOB

A courier delivered my biopsy slides from the urologist's hospital to my radiotherapist's hospital. There, a pathologist classified them a Gleason 3 plus 3, the same total as before. When my slides were returned to the first hospital, they got lost. I never knew whether to blame the hospital or the courier service.

While they were missing, I became agitated. I was already aggravated, and this escalated my exasperation. Wherever I went for treatment, I'd need those slides with me. The thought of having another biopsy horrified me.

But my biopsy slides were found, to my relief, and I had another pathologist read them. He is an old friend and had dealt with prostate cancer himself. I called him when I got home Wednesday afternoon.

"Bob, I read them as a 3 plus 2," he said.

"That's better," I said, but thought it wasn't as good as a 2 plus 2 which my radiotherapist friend would treat with seeds only.

"I wish my slides had looked the way yours do when I was diagnosed,."

"Thanks," I said.

"And a PSA of 3.7. That's still normal."

"Yes, but it jumped from 2.2 to 3.7 in sixteen months."

"I wouldn't advise this in many cases," he said, "but I think you ought to watch and wait."

"No. I need to do something definite."

"That's up to you. But watch and wait is what I'd do for now if it were me."

"But it's me, not you. Look, will you do me a favor?"

"Sure."

"Send my slides by overnight Fed-Ex to Jonathan Epstein at Johns Hopkins."

"I'll do it."

Dr. Jonathan Epstein was a pathologist whose skill at ranking Gleason's score had made him famous.

John and Nancy called from Denver that evening. They had been packing up their Arizona home which they'd sold. Two homes were too much responsibility. John was seventy-eight, and Nancy, in her early sixties.

I wondered how they had kept two houses running for so long. We sold Snuggery Farm because two households involved too much work. Especially since one of them was a seventy-acre property.

Nancy and Saralee listened on phone extensions, so the four of us could chat together, a usual practice for us. John was frank in telling me about his cancer and how he had decided to treat it. This was a review, because John and I had discussed his decision before.

"I've read so much medical information my head is spinning. " I said. "I still can't decide which treatment to choose."

"That happened with me, too. It happens with all of us. Deciding which treatment is right for you is difficult."

"Yes," Saralee agreed. "And Bob wants to decide immediately, if not sooner."

"Bob, do you remember Pat, who assisted me when I was Provost at Marquette?" John asked.

"Vaguely."

"Well, I want you to get in touch with him. He's had prostate cancer, too. Like you, he did a lot of research before making up his mind."

"Okay."

"I'm also going to send you a book about prostate cancer. It's written by a doctor, but it's aimed at the public."

"Fine. Thanks."

"The book is primarily for you, Saralee," Nancy said.

"He's got me reading medical stuff, too," Saralee said. "I'm overwhelmed."

"Whatever you do, don't baby him," Nancy advised.

"Bob, I want to give you the name of the radiation oncologist that I decided to use in Denver."

John gave me his office phone number, too.

"When we interviewed him, Nancy told him we still like to make love when we feel like it."

"I felt brazen, but I had to know," Nancy said.

"I know exactly how you feel," Saralee said to her.

"Part of the reason we chose my doctor was because we trusted him. We felt at ease with him," John said. "Choose someone you feel that way about."

"I'll try," I said.

"I want you to feel free to call Nancy and me anytime. We want to help any way we can."

"Yes," Nancy said. "We should be easy to find, too. We'll be here forever unpacking boxes from Arizona."

"We will stay in touch and keep you in our prayers. Meanwhile, keep the faith. You will beat this."

When we hung up the phone, Saralee asked, "What do you think Nancy meant by not babying you?"

"I'm not sure. Maybe she meant during the treatment or afterwards. If I feel lousy, and you feel sorry for me," I said.

"I'd feel miserable. I sure hope that doesn't happen."

My brother, Howard, called and said, "Call Stan Weinberg. He's got prostate cancer and treated it with something called seeds. What are they?"

"Seeds are radioactive pellets that get shot into the prostate gland to burn it out," I said. "None of the rest of the pelvis gets radiated. It's a less extreme form of treatment than external beam radiation and much less extreme than radical surgery."

"I don't understand all that, but call Stan anyhow. He's smart."

My brother and I don't talk long on the phone, but we do talk frequently. I usually call him. When Howard initiates the call, he has something important to say. I planned to call Stan soon.

SARALEE

Sometimes, Bob gets telephonitis. He set a new record on Thursday.

I retreated to my library to write this book. Our libraries are two rooms away, so I can't hear his constant calls. I can't hear much of anything when I'm writing. My concentration is total. Nothing exists except what's spilling out of my mind through the keyboard and onto the computer screen.

He decided to call his medical school car pool. He remembered them as being the best and the brightest, not plodders like himself.

First, Bob tried to find Alan's number. He had no record of it, nor did telephone information. Alan was a medical oncologist, probably part of an oncology group. That would explain why his name wasn't listed separately. His home phone was unlisted, too.

Then, he called Phil at home. He'd already left for the office or the hospital. His wife, Betty, told Bob that she would find Phil and have him call. Betty knew Alan's office number and gave it to Bob.

Alan told Bob to avoid surgery. It was a gory operation. The complications afterwards were enormous. Bob told Alan his PSA and that only one of six biopsy cores was involved, and that one minimally.

Alan suggested that Bob opt for the least invasive treatment—as little as possible. And that he need be in no hurry to make any decision. Time was on his side.

Bob called my cousin in California, also a medical oncologist, and told him what Alan had said. Larry agreed with Alan's assessment. He told Bob to stay cool. Not to panic.

Bob called the pathologist who had initially read his Gleason as a 3 plus 3. He told him that another pathologist at his hospital had read it as a 3 plus 2. The pathologist said that the two readings were nearly identical.

Bob called Dr. Epstein. He had read the biopsy slides as a 3 plus 3. Bob asked him what treatment he would recommend for himself or his father. He said that he'd choose surgery. Of course. Dr. Epstein was at Johns Hopkins where Dr. Patrick Walsh was the pro-surgery director of the urology department. Bob asked Dr. Epstein to send his slides back to the hospital in Atlanta. He promised he would.

Bob called John's radiation therapist in Denver who told Bob that there were many choices available with a Gleason 6 or even with a Gleason 7. He recommended external beam followed by seeds.

Bob called George, a mutual friend from Emory. George had opted for radical surgery and complained about the post-surgical follow-up. His PSA was 15. His doctors had told him they were not sure of the significance of PSA testing. He sounded very ill at ease.

I came out of my library a few times for coffee. Bob was always on the phone. He kept me up to date on his conversations. Along with the medical calls, he kept phoning for all sorts of investment information, and the faxes kept rolling in. He was a very busy boy.

Bob called Stan Weinberg in Pittsburgh. Stan told him he had done six months of independent research and plenty of doctor consultations. He decided on seed implantation and had it done four months ago. He felt great. Stan told Bob that he had lots of erections, more than before surgery. But he had nothing to do with them. Stan lived alone with no romantic attachments. He was seventy-one and a confirmed bachelor.

Phil called and said he wanted to talk to both of us.

"Phil, I'm in big trouble," Bob said.

Bob explained his problem, the numbers, the choices. Phil was an internist, and we expected a generalist's positive opinion from him. What we got was extremely conservative.

"I think, with proper treatment, it is likely you will be cured," Phil said.

I walked into Bob's study. He has a large desk, a pub table that I once gave him as a birthday present. Today it was covered with prostate-cancer articles, Bob's test results, and faxes.

"I think I'm going to try Zeke," Bob said.

"Okay. May I speak to him when you're done?" I asked.

"Sure."

Zeke was a pathologist and the brightest of the car pool. He'd always been my favorite of those guys. Both witty and handsome, he was a winner.

Bob found Zeke at the hospital. I left his study to give him privacy. Calling the car pool was a trip down memory lane; I'd allow him time to reminisce. I'd let him do whatever he needed to make this difficult decision.

I craved moderation. A minimal treatment plan. I wanted to tell him that. But I didn't dare. What if I were wrong?

When Bob was finished talking with Zeke, he called, "Saralee, Zeke wants to talk to you."

I sat on our bed and picked up the phone.

"Hello, Zeke," I said.

"Hi, Saralee. Sorry about all this."

"Me, too. He's driving us both crazy trying to decide how to treat his cancer."

"He has so little of it."

"I know. He's terribly upset and not always rational. Forgive him if he sounds extreme."

"He seems unduly upset."

"Yes. What did you tell him?"

"About all the options of treatment."

"All of them? Including those that are least harmful?"

"Yes."

"Like what?" I asked.

"Like maybe a little hormonal treatment if he thought that would make him feel more in charge of the deal."

"Do you think he needs that?"

"No, I told him watchful waiting would be fine."

"What did he say to that?"

"He didn't want to hear that."

"I know. He's determined to over-treat himself."

"That's what I gathered."

"And I'm going to let him do that. Even if he decides on radical prostatectomy."

"He's not likely to opt for that, is he?"

"I don't know. He vacillates. It's hard to know what he's thinking."

"He sounds unfocused."

"He is. Nonetheless, Bob's got to make his own decision. Because if its a bad decision, he's going to die angry. I don't want him to die angry at me."

"I understand."

"I like happy campers."

"I told him he could wait three months and have another PSA," Zeke said. "They can fluctuate. Then, if it's still 3.7, he could have another biopsy."

"What did he think of that?"

"Not much. There's such a thing as false positive, too."

"I don't think he's dealing with a false positive. His PSA has gone up quickly, and his biopsy result is positive."

"Yes."

"Zekey, do you still have tons of curly blond hair? Are you still tall, lean, and handsome?"

"Somewhat less so," he said and laughed. "What do you look like?"

"I have the shortest head of hair you've ever seen, and it's grey, almost white. I probably look more glamorous than I did when we were all young. But I'm old. I'll be sixty in May."

"That's okay. What do you do for yourself?"

"I write."

"What do you write?"

"Poetry and prose. I've published dozens of poems and some short prose. My first prose book is being considered by two publishing houses. One of them is in San Francisco."

"When you come here for your book signing, we'll go to dinner."

"I'm a long way from a book signing. The publishers are only reading two stories from the book. They haven't even requested the whole manuscript yet."

"Good luck."

"Thanks, I'll need it. In numerous ways."

"Yes, goodbye."

"'Bye."

I hung up the phone, and tears sprang to my eyes. Bob was in his study, so he couldn't see. I cried very quietly, so he couldn't hear either. We had all been so invincible and immortal, back in the carpool days.

All the calls Bob made that day still left us in limbo, stranded, lost in a void.

Bob worked as usual on Friday. When he got home, I could

sense his tension. A boring hour-and-a-half drive each way provides lots of time to juggle alternatives.

"I think I ought to have surgery," he said.

"Why?"

"It's the 'gold standard'."

"What's that supposed to mean?"

"It has a longer track record. They've been doing it longer."

"Oh."

"I might just as well retire before they operate."

"That's crazy."

"No, it isn't. Where will I get coverage for the weeks I'm out of commission?"

"Jim could work for you more than just Mondays and Thursdays. He'd be delighted with the extra income."

"What about Fridays?"

Jim worked at another hospital on Friday.

"Art has worked a couple of Fridays for you. If you ask him in advance, I bet he'll cover Fridays until you're well enough to work again."

"That'll be five or six weeks. Will my staff doctors still be loyal to me?"

"I certainly hope so. You've been with them for eleven years now."

"Look at Addison. He's retired. He seems perfectly happy."

"Ad still does consulting work."

Bob spread prostate cancer articles on his desk and put his head in his hands. I left his study quietly.

I sensed the start of a difficult weekend. He'd bounce from surgery to external beam, from external beam that included seeding, from seeding alone, then back to surgery. He'd alternate talking with silence, while he brooded.

I phoned the Luces. Piera answered.

"May I come to your apartment?" I asked.

"Yes, sure," Piera said.

"Right now?"

"Of course."

I rode the elevator four floors. Ad opened the door, and Piera kissed me.

"I need a place to hide for a while. Bob keeps changing his mind. At the moment, he favors surgery."

"That's an established way of treating prostate cancer," Ad said.

"I'm afraid of the surgery itself and of the complications afterwards. But I can't say that to him."

"Why?" Piera said.

"Because if he makes a bad decision based on what I say, he'll hate me."

"Well, you don't have to make the decision. But you should be able to tell him what you think and express how you feel," Ad said.

"He says he wants to retire like you, Ad. I told him you do consulting work."

"Tell him I don't think this is the right moment to retire," Ad said.

"Tell him yourself. He's rereading cancer articles at his desk right now. He may bury himself in them all weekend."

"Yes?"

"He keeps ricochetting off the walls, changing his mind. If he'd stop bouncing around, I could settle down, too."

"Yes, but he's trying to decide what's best," Ad said.

"All right. I need a place to cry."

I walked to an interior corner of their living room, faced it, and tried to cry. Nothing happened. I felt so boxed in, physically and emotionally.

"Saralee, go to our bedroom," Piera said. "Close the door. Sit in a comfortable chair. Relax. Let the tears come."

I did that, but no tears came. Although sitting in their peaceful bedroom relaxed me. When I rode the elevator back home and opened our front door, I could focus on Bob's dilemma again.

BOB

It's a tough call to make. What to do about prostate cancer. No form of treatment is without risk. I had taught Saralee enough for her to become devil's advocate.

If I was surgery-minded, she'd say, "You couldn't tolerate being cut from the belly button to the pubic bone. You've never had major surgery. The most pain you've ever dealt with was in the dentist's chair."

"I can tolerate anything that will get rid of this cancer permanently."

"There's no assuredness that surgery will do that."

"More assuredness than with any other treatment."

"Highest rate of impotence and incontinence. Stress incontinence guaranteed."

When I considered external beam, she'd say, "That burns up the entire area. You can't have surgery in the pelvis afterwards."

"You mean more cancer surgery?"

"No. There are other things that can go wrong. Non-cancerous things that require surgery. All you think about is cancer."

"Because that's what I have. That's what I'm fighting."

"External beam has almost as high a risk for impotence as surgery without the track record of surgery."

"How about external beam and seeds?"

"Both? You have so damn little cancer. That's overkill."

When I considered seeds alone, she'd say, "That has the shortest track record of them all."

"What is it that you advise, my consultant?"

"I can't advise anything. You're the one who's got to decide. It's your body."

Later that night she put her arms around me and said, "We've got to salvage something out of all this grief. An increased awareness of how much we love each other. Of how glorious our life together has been and can be again."

"If I'm lucky."

"But a life we'll appreciate more because of what we're living through now."

"Yes."

She's so much more articulate than I.

SARALEE

We had dinner with Carrie and Rogers, support-team members, at our apartment on Saturday. Carrie is the curator of modern and contemporary art at the High Museum. We bonded when I did research on their Joseph Cornell collection, eleven works given to the High by the Cornell Foundation.

Rogers is the husband Carrie spirited away from his successful real estate company in Tallahassee, Florida, where he had always lived. He and Bob share a natural affinity for one another.

Bob would make his mushroom risotto, and I would steam fish. I helped Bob cut up the fresh mushrooms, rehydrate the dry ones, chop herbs, and prepare mushroom and chicken broth for his risotto. We're a good cooking team.

When Carrie and Rogers arrived, Bob would stir and add, stir and add, until his *arborio* rice was plump and creamy. Rogers would sit at the counter, and they would relate.

My steelhead trout was a no-brainer. I'd seasoned and covered it with a plastic bag, then I'd put it in the microwave and set the timer. Rogers would push the start button and call us when the rice was almost done.

We left the men in the kitchen and went to my library. Carrie and I sat on opposite ends of my sofa.

"This is a terrible time for us," I said.

"You're not making things any better by dwelling on what's terrible," she answered. "Look outside. It's a beautiful day."

"Yes, it's beautiful out there, but it's not beautiful here," I said and pointed at myself.

"Well, you need to focus on what's beautiful and let that inform you."

"We're both miserable."

"You don't have to be. Bob isn't in the slightest bit of pain. He can take all the time he wants to make his decision."

"He insists the decision be made quickly."

"Then let him do that."

"He's not exactly rational right now."

"Neither are you."

"You're right. I did the craziest thing last week."

"Like what?"

"I bought a boneless leg of lamb on sale at the new A&P and an eye of the round roast on sale at Harris Teeter and put them in my freezer. Each one weighs five pounds. We'll never eat five pounds of meat before it spoils."

"Why did you do that?"

"I thought the roasts would make me feel safer."

"Did they make you feel safer?"

"No, stupider."

"Take the roasts back and have them cut in half."

"That's a great idea. Why didn't I think of that?"

"Because you're not thinking straight. The four of us are together to share our friendship, to celebrate with a great meal. Focus on that."

"I'll try."

"It's a beautiful day. There's not a single thing wrong with today. Let's talk about Picasso."

Carrie is hard at work on the Picasso exhibition, a loan from the Museum of Modern Art in New York. She and a curator from MOMA have collaborated on the exhibit. Picasso would open in a few weeks; its installation took all her time. She had generously put time aside for us.

Thoroughly animated, Carrie talked about opening crates to find delightful surprises inside. Her red hair glistened and her green eyes gleamed, as she described the pleasure of opening the "gifts,"as she called the MOMA loans, and then deciding where to hang them. Time flew, until Rogers called us to dinner.

Rogers asked to say grace. We all bowed our heads and folded our hands. It was a simple prayer that ended with, "We thank you, Lord, for allowing us to share this day. It's a beautiful day."

"It's a beautiful day" became a new mantra for Bob and me.

BOB

Monday's mail brought a letter from John's friend, Pat. He explained how he had dealt with his prostate cancer. He had done his own research, and, at fifty-four, he had opted for surgery. The letter was both formal and frank.

He wrote, "In choosing a surgeon, I set up a template to evaluate the surgeon. The most important factors were number of procedures performed in a month (you want someone who does a lot of them); the average time of surgery; the average amount of blood used during the procedure; and any outcome data they might be able to share.

"The enclosed article was the most helpful in developing a perspective on the process. There is no need to return it."

The article, published in *Fortune* magazine, was entitled "Taking on Prostate Cancer" and had been written by Andy Grove, the CEO of Intel. He was diagnosed with prostate cancer at age fifty-eight with a PSA of 5. He thought of his tumor as a sugar cube. When his PSA rose, he realized that his sugar cube was growing.

An extremely intelligent man with no medical education, Andy Grove had done his own medical research anyhow. He learned that most doctors published their own data without comparing it to the data of others publishing in the same field. He was forced to do his own cross-comparisons. I admired his intellect and persistence.

A radiotherapist told him about "smart bomb" radiation. Highly radioactive seeds are momentarily inserted into the gland through wire-like tubes and then the wires and seeds are removed. Local anesthesia is used.

The doctor called external beam radiation "carpet bombing," because it exposed neighboring organs, such as the rectum and urethra, to radiation. Smart bomb radiation would cut down the amount of carpet bomb therapy.

Grove said, "It sounded like an elegant alternative to surgery. I asked that doctor, 'If you had what I have, what would you do?' He said, 'I would probably have surgery.' I left, utterly confused."

He had an ultrasound done at a university hospital with an elaborate new-fangled machine. It showed a 60% chance that the cancer extended beyond the prostate gland. Using a Johns Hopkins graph, he reached the same conclusion.

He did research on the recurrence rate of cancer. PSA had been around for only ten years, so he concluded that both surgery and radiation could offer relevant data for ten years or less.

Andy Grove took nine months to reach a decision, nine months of research and doctor consultations. In all, he talked to fifteen physicians and half a dozen patients. I admired his thoroughness.

Urologists qualified his tumor as a T2a or a T2b. His Gleason score was 7. He watched his PSA climb from 5 to 6. Andy Grove needed to act.

On a biking trip, he unwound and made a decision. He would have smart bomb radiation followed by external beam. For smart bombs, he went to a doctor in Seattle.

Seattle. That word kept cropping up. My Atlanta urologist had said the best radiation data was in Seattle. My radiotherapist here had talked about the implant work that Dr. John Blasko was doing in Seattle. Andy Grove had gone to Seattle for treatment with a "smart bomb" doctor. I looked through my pile of medical articles. I found three articles John Blasko had authored; in two, his was the lead name. I needed to talk with Blasko.

On Monday afternoon I tried to call him at Northwest Hospital, the address on his medical articles. I was told that he was no longer there and was given the name of the clinic where he practiced now. I called and spoke with his secretary, who said they had been lucky to lure Dr. Blasko to their clinic. He said that Dr. Blasko was diffi-cult to reach, but I should keep trying.

I tried four times, and I finally reached him on Tuesday evening from my motel room. I told Dr. Blasko my statistics and test results. He said that I sounded like a candidate for seed implantation, peri-od. External beam plus seeding would be overkill. I was elated.

I phoned Saralee and said, "I found him. I talked to Blasko. I told him all about my numbers and tests."

"What did he say?"

"To do seeds only. That external beam and seeds would be too much treatment. He called it 'overkill' just like you did."

"What do you think about that?"

"I have to think it through."

"Okay, sweet dreams. I love you."

"I love you, too. When we're together again tomorrow afternoon, we'll talk."

Saralee called me at the hospital the next morning and said, "For a guy who likes easy rolls, you sure are making this hard."

That's a joke between us. As a kid going out to dinner with my family, I was once asked if I wanted a hard or soft roll. I said that I wanted an easy roll. I do like easy rolls. That's my style.

"You're right," I said. "I guess we're going to Seattle."

On Wednesday afternoon Saralee and I called the clinic in Seattle and spoke with Dr. Blasko's scheduling secretary. I asked for an appointment with Dr. Blasko. She said that they needed my records for Dr. Blasko to evaluate before any appointment could be made.

"I'll fax all of them to you," I said. "How soon can he see me?"

"There's one appointment open on December 4th, but I can't book you until Dr. Blasko has had time to evaluate the information you send," she said.

"Can't you just pencil my name in lightly?"

"Sorry, no. And that's just the first appointment. We'll do tests on you here and plan an individualized implant scheme. You'll come a second time for surgery."

"Why do we have to come to Seattle twice?" Saralee asked. "Why can't you do the tests and surgery on the same trip?"

"Because it takes time to do the plan and more time to get the seeds. You need to travel here twice."

She explained that I would have a volume study by ultrasound to show the shape of my prostate and a pelvic arch CT during the consultation.

A pelvic arch CT shows the placement of the prostate in relation to the pelvis. If the pubic bone lies in front of the prostate, you can't use the regulated template to place seeds evenly. The needles used with the template can't go through bone.

The surgery would take place three to six weeks after the consultation. I would be in Seattle the day before the seed implantation surgery. On the day after it, I would be seen by a nurse and a resident. I could fly back to Atlanta the day after that. My local urologist would do any necessary follow-up.

I faxed all my information immediately.

I tried to find Dr. Blasko on Friday without success. I tried again on Monday. I got his appointments secretary instead. She told me Dr. Blasko had reviewed my information. I was a candidate for seed implantation. The earliest appointment was Monday, December 15.

I asked to speak to Dr. Blasko. She said that he was unavailable. I booked the appointment and asked when I could speak with him. Surely, he would find an earlier time to see a fellow doctor. She said that I needed to catch him between cases, but he was very busy and very tired. I tried several more times and finally got lucky.

Dr. Blasko sounded harassed. He couldn't see me sooner. He told me that if he worked any harder, he could have a heart attack. Saralee told him she wouldn't want that to happen to him. I explained how anxious I felt about carrying this cancer inside me and how scared that it would grow or metastasize.

He said, "What about Ragde?"

Dr. Haakon Ragde was the urologist Dr. Blasko had worked with at Northwest Hospital. In all the articles that I had read about Seattle and seed implantation, Dr. Haakon Ragde was an author. On one, his name appeared as lead author. I hunted him up on the Internet. He had done over 2000 implants.

Saralee and I called Dr. Ragde's office. Because someone had canceled his appointment, Dr. Ragde could see me on Friday, October 4th. A volume study to determine the size and shape of my prostate gland would be done then, too. I would also meet with Dr. Robert Meier, who would be my radiotherapist.

We grabbed the appointment with an enormous sense of relief. I had made my decision. We could back our way out of hell and see the pure light of day again. From now on, I vowed we would make every day beautiful.

SARALEE

It was only four days until we'd leave on vacation. I swung into action and made travel arrangements for Seattle, three days after our return. I called the club line, a toll-free telephone number that makes hotel reservations for the Club Corporation of America. They booked us at the Hotel Vintage Park in downtown Seattle at a reduced rate. I called Delta and found that they provided the only non-stop service between Atlanta and Seattle.

"Grab all your frequent flyer miles, and let's go to Delta's ticket office," I said.

"I don't think we have enough Delta frequent flyer miles for free tickets," Bob said.

"Then take all your American Express miles, too."

We drove to the Delta ticket office a few blocks away and parked in a fifteen minute spot reserved for plane reservations. We'd need to fly to Seattle on Thursday in order to be there for Friday morning appointments. We could fly back on the Friday night red-eye, but neither of us felt up for that. We'd fly back on Saturday.

"If you spend one more night in Seattle and leave on Sunday, the rate is $343 a person," the sales agent told us. "Otherwise, it's $1144."

"We'll be recovering from a six-hour time change. We won't want to stay in Seattle long enough to adjust to an additional three-hour change," I said. "We'll use frequent flyer miles."

"That's another way of doing it," the agent said.

She booked reservations for us. Since we didn't have enough Delta miles, she gave us the forms to convert American Express miles to Delta and told us the swiftest way to make the conversion.

Even so, our timing would be close. We had to hope the conversion miles would be in the mail when we got back home from vacation, so we could pick up our free tickets at Delta.

We went to The Temple on Wednesday evening and Thursday morning for Rosh Hashanah services celebrating the Jewish New Year. I prayed that the decision we had come to was right. We needed God's blessing to begin this new year.

BOB

We drove to the hospital to pick up my biopsy slides after temple on Thursday. We'd take them to Seattle with us. Saralee had nagged me to pick up everything, all the unused portions of the biopsy cores, too.

"I don't know much about medicine, but I know lots about being a patient," she said.

"Meaning what?" I said.

"Meaning that you need to keep your records in your own hands. You'll take better care of them than anyone else."

When we got home, I opened the insulated bag cushioning my slides. In it were three of the nine slides that had been sent to Johns Hopkins. Irate, I called the pathology department at Johns Hopkins and spoke to a histology technician. She told me that they could not locate the other six slides.

"How can you lose something this important?" I yelled.

"They have to be here somewhere," she said.

"Have you checked Dr. Epstein's office?"

"The door is locked, but I'll check there."

"You've got to find my slides. I need them for Seattle."

"I'll do my best. Sometimes slides get put on another tray. Sometimes Dr. Epstein keeps them in his office. I'll keep looking."

I called Jonathan Epstein's office and left a message on his voice mail. I adopted a composure that I didn't feel.

"I need my slides for a consultation in Seattle," I said. "Will you please help locate them?"

I doubted he'd be available that day. Like me, he was celebrating Rosh Hashanah. I wanted him to know that my slides had been lost.

I envisioned myself needing another biopsy. Would it be better to have the local urologist do that right now or to wait until we got back home? Right now, probably. A biopsy on Monday in Atlanta and a volume study on Friday in Seattle would invite infection.

After a wait that seemed endless, the technician called and said that she had found my six slides. They had been put on a tray where they didn't belong. She apologized and offered to send them to me by Fed-Ex overnight. I thanked her.

SARALEE

We packed. Mostly, we down-sized the amount of clothes we intended to take. Bob, who planned on three pairs of shoes, packed one pair of loafers. He'd wear his rubber-bottomed shoes most of the time. He packed a sport coat, some trousers, and a suit, with one shirt and tie. I packed a black suit that has both slacks and a skirt, a textured jacket, and a pair of taupe slacks. We each took a few sweaters. We had never traveled for ten days with bags so light.

We had promised each other we'd leave Bob's prostate gland in Atlanta. We had agreed the "C" word wouldn't be mentioned. It wasn't. Whatever thoughts of cancer that crept in remained nonverbalized.

It's easy to lose yourself in Italy. The gracious old hotels. The fabulous food. The autostrada where Bob drove like an Italian speed demon in the far-left lane. The country roads winding through hilly vineyards and villages. Ideal weather, except for a shower while we ate lunch in Barolo. Venice, the most beautiful city we've ever seen.

We lost our way continually during the trip. Accommodating Italians set us straight. We were directed in Italian with sign language and sometimes in immaculate English. People put us on the right route by letting us follow their cars. Once, a man on a bicycle led us to a needed road. A farmer in a tiny three-wheeled truck guided us back and through a turn we had overlooked. In Venice, a woman put her hand under my elbow and took us from a square onto the street we sought. We must have looked as fragile as we felt.

I had some diarrhea while we were away. I frequently do when we travel. I look at it as a win/win proposition. I can eat anything I want and not gain weight. The calories don't stick around long enough to convert into fat. On the last day I felt a tickle in my throat. I had a cold.

Our flight arrived in Atlanta early, and we were home by 3:30. Bob hunted anxiously through our mail and found the conversion miles that we needed to pick up our frequent flyer tickets from Delta.

Bob checked our voice mail and found seven messages. He erased all of them except those for me. He seemed upset.

"What's wrong?" I asked.

"Dr. Ragde called while we were gone. He said I was a candidate for seed implantation."

"That's great."

"No it isn't. He doesn't know I'm coming there this week."

"When was the message left?"

"I don't remember."

"Bob, Dr. Ragde hasn't been told when you're scheduled. Your appointment for Friday hasn't been canceled."

"I'm going to call Ragde's office to make sure."

"Suit yourself."

I didn't tell him then how annoyed I was that he had erased Dr. Ragde's message before I heard it. I had shouldered the grief with him and deserved to share any benefits. Later, I had that out with him.

"The office is closed," he agonized after calling Dr. Ragde's office.

I looked at my watch and said, "Naturally, it's closed. It's lunch time in Seattle."

"We can't pick up our tickets at Delta until I'm sure he's going to see me."

"Okay. You finish opening your mail. I'm taking some clothes to the cleaners, so we can pack them for Seattle freshly pressed. By the time I get back, you'll have this resolved. We'll go to Delta together."

Pulling back into our garage, I saw ripe tomatoes on our three plants. I picked seven. They'd please our palates and perk up our spirits.

Decision

~

BOB

OCTOBER 16–18, 1997

The Seattle Experience: that's what one journal article called it. We had both agreed that Seattle was the right choice for me. We both jumped at the opportunity for this early appointment.

We both knew that we would fly to Seattle on Thursday morning after arriving home on Monday from a fourteen-hour trip with a six-hour time change. We both realized that we'd still have residual jet-lag when we reached Seattle and added another three-hour time change.

What we hadn't counted on was Saralee's cold which was miserable on Thursday morning. I brought her a glass of my fresh-squeezed orange juice which she downed with her usual Plaquenil, plus two aspirins and a Claritin to clear her sinuses.

"I feel lousy," she said. "My voice sounds hoarse now, and by mid-afternoon I'll sound like a frog. The same way I've sounded since Monday, like the transformed diva in 'Phantom of the Opera.'"

"I know. Maybe hot coffee will help."

"I can't taste a thing. Your coffee will be wasted on me."

I brought her a mug anyhow. She tilted her head back and

dripped Afrin into each nostril.

"I can hardly breathe. My left nostril is completely blocked."

"Drink some coffee."

"I have more diarrhea now than during our vacation. We shouldn't take short trips with big time changes. Two weeks with weekends on both sides would be better."

"You have a point there. We'll stay longer next time."

"That'll be easier on our systems. Mine in particular, because lupus screwed up my immune system. My idiotic body refuses to move. Why the heck do we have to go to Seattle today?"

"Because my appointment is tomorrow morning, a volume survey at 10:30, a meeting with Dr. Ragde at 1:15, and a meeting with Dr. Meier at 2:00. You really don't have to go with me."

"What sort of baloney is that, partner?"

"It's the truth. I can handle this on my own."

"Fat chance," she said.

Saralee drank a mug of coffee, and I brought her a second one.

"Why did we take this appointment?" she asked.

"Honey, this was the only appointment he had for weeks to come. Somebody canceled, and I was given his appointment. I'm a work-in."

I don't know why she didn't remember that. She had listened on the phone when I made the appointment.

"Look, Saralee, you can stay here. In bed. Comfortable. I'll call you all the time and tell you how things are going."

As answer, she flung off the bed covers and crossed to her sink to floss and brush her teeth. I went to my bathroom to do the same.

I shaved and dressed in the clothes she had put aside for me, a black knit shirt and plaid slacks. By the time I returned to our bedroom, she had dressed, made the bed, and put the finishing touches on her make-up.

"You look great," I said.

She did. She had on black slacks, a black sweater, and a brightly striped tunic. Even her loafers and handbag matched, that woven leather stuff. She's a dresser. I like that about her.

"I feel crappy."

"Don't go."

As answer, she picked up her canvas bag and my umbrella. I put my carry-on bag over one shoulder and our shared garment bag in the other hand.

In that garment bag, she had packed my frequently lost biopsy slides and my MRI, both of which were too wide for our canvas bags. We would carry our luggage onto the airplane. That way, nothing could be lost.

She had done our packing the day before. She usually folds my dress shirts, and I pack for myself. When I got home from my hospital on Wednesday afternoon and unloaded my shaving kit, she showed me exactly where it fit in the bag that I'd take to Seattle.

She's usually a good kid. She really felt awful that morning, and her cold was the least of it. We were both scared and nervous.

SARALEE

The Buckhead Safety Cab was waiting at our building's front door. The driver loaded our bags into the trunk, and Bob draped our garment bag, with his MRI and his biopsy slides, carefully on top.

"We're headed for the airport, Delta," Bob said. Take Interstate 400."

"Atlanta is staging its own version of the Million Man March this morning. You can't move on 400. The interstates are parking lots all the way downtown."

Another example that nothing would go smoothly for us. I had scant hope our luck would change.

"What time is your flight?" he asked.

"10:57, but we already have our tickets and aren't checking luggage."

It was 9:30 now.

"I'll get you there on time. But in order to avoid traffic, I'll use an unconventional route."

To call his route unconventional was British understatement. He traveled through an odd conglomeration of streets to get us past the marchers downtown. Then he took the freeway to the airport. As he drove, he told us about retiring, getting bored, and opting to drive a cab. We arrived at the airport by 10:05.

Bob has a senior citizen's card that entitles him to a 20% discount on taxi fares in Atlanta. He didn't use the card. Instead, he tipped generously.

We boarded our plane on time, then sat around on the tarmac. The captain kept repeating that Delta's computer system had been inadvertently shut down. We would leave any minute, as soon as it booted up again.

The plane backed out thirty-five minutes late, taxied down the runway, and waited in line for its turn to take off. Four and a half hours' travel had been increased to over five hours by the delay.

We had reserved seats on adjacent aisles. Bob's set of three seats held only Bob. A row behind us, a set of three seats was entirely vacant. I moved there. We raised the arms between seats, settled cushions against the windows, put up our feet, and covered our legs with blankets. I pulled down my window shade to close out the world. I tried to read *The Satanic Verses*.

I'm moved by Salman Rushdie's writing, its density and complexity. He's the best author that I've read since Shakespeare, maybe even better. That's going some for a Shakespeare scholar.

In a single paragraph, Rushdie can hurl you into tragedy while tickling you with belly laughs. The book begins with Gibreel and Saladin plummeting from an exploded jet plane to the sea with no more parachute than each other to cling to. The fall is tragic, but the way Gibreel commands Saladin to learn how to fly is comic. I read slowly, because I wanted this book to last forever.

Each time I looked up from my book, reality rushed in. You can't close the world out by pulling down a window shade. I dreaded what might be ahead for the two of us—Bob's body, our lives.

I ate fruit and yogurt and drank canned water that tasted metallic, then napped briefly. I blew my nose incessantly, drizzled nose drops, took aspirins, and sucked a few Halls mentho-lyptus drops. When the pilot announced we could see Mount Rainier from my side of the plane, I didn't raise my window shade to look.

I returned to my assigned seat as the fasten-your-seat-belt sign came on and a stewardess announced that we were making our initial descent into Seattle. The window shade beside me was up, and the mountains looked awesome.

"It sure is gorgeous," I croaked.

The man beside the window nodded and smiled. It was the first time I had spoken in over four hours. My laryngitis seemed slightly less prominent. I hoped that I wouldn't sound like a frog when we met with the doctors tomorrow.

BOB

We had left cloudy Atlanta with its forecast of rain and arrived in sunny Seattle. It was balmy, almost hot.

"Do you have air-conditioning?" I asked the taxi driver as we sped toward downtown.

"Yes," he said, "but it's not working."

"Saralee, this cab has been imported from Atlanta," I said.

Atlanta cabbies often claim that they have air-conditioning, but it's temporarily broken. She grinned, then laughed. It was hard to be glum on such a beautiful day.

"Look," I said, "There's the Space Needle they put up for the 1962 World's Fair."

I was holding her hand. We've done a lot of hand holding in the last few months.

"How do you know they put it up in '62?"

"I've been reading *Access Seattle,* the book you gave me on the plane. You told me that you'd bought the book, made our hotel and dinner reservations, and packed our bags. So it was my job to plan this afternoon's activity."

"What did you plan?"

"We're going to SAM."

"What's Sam?"

"The Seattle Art Museum. The people here call it SAM. It's only a few blocks from the hotel."

"SAM sounds fine to me. We haven't been in Seattle for over twenty years."

"Yes, we stayed for three days. The sky was always blue. The sun always shined."

"People said it was a miracle. Three sunny days in a row."

We arrived at the Hotel Vintage Park. The hotel looked elegant—old, small, and well decorated.

The clerk at the reception desk told us that check-out time was one o'clock and check-in time was four. Rooms were available on the fourth and tenth floors.

"Is either vacant?" Saralee asked.

"Both are vacant, but neither has been cleaned yet. I can't promise you a clean room until 4:00, but we'll be happy to store your luggage until then."

"Are they both on the Spring Street side of the hotel?" I asked.

"Yes," the receptionist said.

"Good. That's the quiet side of the hotel. Which room do you prefer, Saralee?"

"The one on the tenth floor. How did you know the Spring Street side was quieter?"

"*Access Seattle*," I said and felt perky that I knew.

Saralee usually plans our trips and pays attention to fine details. This trip had been planned hastily. She hadn't time for details such as where the quietest rooms could be found.

"Wait here while I check something."

She went through a doorway marked "Tulio" and returned with a menu in her hand.

"The restaurant looks great," she said. "Northern Italian food, all the stuff we adore."

I took the menu from her but said nothing.

"I feel scrambled—too long in the air, too much time change, too much anxiety and despair."

"Yes," I agreed.

"It would be civilized to sit down at a table and have a bite to eat. We needn't order much."

"Okay."

"The people inside are mostly upscale business types, women in tailored suits, men in ties and jackets. We'll look a little seedy, but who cares."

The hostess gave us a window table. With sunshine obscuring my vision, I pulled the curtains shut. In no time flat, we were sipping wine and ordering—pasta for me and a salad for her. The manager came to be sure the food pleased us. We assured him it did.

"Seattle looks beautiful today," I said.

The manager parted the curtains, looked out, and smiled.

"It's days like this that keep us going," he said. "Enjoy your meal."

To my surprise, our room was ready when we finished lunch. We moved in and unpacked our few belongings; the most precious, of course, were my biopsy slides, MRI films, and other test results, plus a few of the medical studies I had read. I knew some of those papers almost by heart, especially one with Dr. Ragde's name as lead author.

We sat side by side on oversized armchairs with our legs and feet propped on equally oversized ottomans. Saralee reached over the table between us and stroked my knee.

"This is not all bad," she said. "We have nothing to do all day except amuse ourselves. It's a vacation day."

"That's true enough."

We say these up-beat things to one another to mask our fear.

"Tomorrow, we'll hop a taxi to Northwest Hospital, you'll have a test, meet your doctors, and set up an appointment for implant surgery soon."

"The sooner the better," I said. "I'm plenty uncomfortable carrying this sucker around. Cancer can grow and spread fast."

"Yes, but we both know prostate cancer is usually slow growing. Let's go out and play."

We stopped at the concierge's desk and Greg, whom Saralee had spoken with by phone, whipped out a map, showed us the route to SAM, and to the spots she had chosen for dinners. All were a few blocks from the hotel.

"You can't miss seeing your dinner destination for tonight," he said. "It's at the top of the Columbia Tower, by far the tallest building in Seattle. When you walk out the hotel door, look left."

"Thanks."

"Save time to drink some wine with me before going to dinner," Greg said. "I pour samples of Washington state wines every evening between 6:00 and 7:00. Tonight, we'll taste a chardonnay and a cabernet sauvignon from Columbia winery."

Greg was personable and friendly with none of the starchiness that I usually associate with a concierge. He set a standard for the friendliness and consideration that we would be shown by numerous Seattleites.

"We'll do that," I said. "New wines are always fun to taste."

Then we headed for SAM, down streets as hilly as those in San Francisco. We held hands as we walked, not so much for balance as for mutual support because of our increased interdependence.

SAM's exterior juxtaposed convex and concave curves. A mammoth black sculpture dominated the court beside the main entrance. As I took money out of my wallet for tickets, Saralee said, "Let's not do this."

"Why?" I asked.

"I caught a glimpse of the waterfront, only a few more blocks downhill. It would be fun to walk along the harbor this balmy afternoon.

"Hopefully we'll return to Seattle soon. We can visit the museum then."

The ticket seller overheard us and said, "That's a good idea. Enjoy our ideal weather. When you get back, our Leonardo da Vinci exhibit will be hung. Visit us then."

Another friendly Seattleite.

SARALEE

We walked down a steep set of steps, under an elevated highway, and stood beside the bay, still holding hands. I needed to touch him—both for security and to show my support.

The dazzling blue water exhilarated us. We watched ferries docking. Passengers left, and passengers boarded. Soon the ferry tooted and left the dock, to be replaced immediately by another ferry.

We stood there a long time and held hands, a quiet meditation that suited both of us. A few days ago, we had found the same satisfaction at the shore of the Adriatic Sea. Today we shared that pleasure by the edge of the Pacific. And pacific was the operative word for our mood.

As we dressed for dinner that night, I said, "I'm sorry I was so nasty this morning."

"It doesn't matter. I'd already forgotten all about it."

"I felt awful, and I didn't remember that your appointment was a work-in, the only one available for weeks."

He crossed the room and held me in his arms. "It's okay, honey. These are rough times for us. Sometimes one or the other of us cracks. I'm glad you're here. I need you so much."

I couldn't begin to express how much I needed him. He's more than half of me. Though it's not psychologically sound, I'm fonder of him than of myself. I'm too hard on me. He's easygoing and accepting—of anything short of cancer.

The Columbia Towers Club was all it should be: sophisticated, elegant, and probably expensive. I don't know exactly how expensive, because I got a guest menu without prices.

I went to the bathroom before dinner. The full moon rose, huge and red as Mars, while I sat in an enclosed stall. This would be my last bout with my unreliable gut, but I didn't know that then.

A woman came into the ladies' and called, "Is anyone here? Do you mind if I show my husband this view of the moon?"

"I'm here," I said, "and I don't mind at all."

When they left and I had finished, I led Bob to the ladies' room and showed him that view of the huge moon rising. From our window table at dinner, we surveyed the city, a patchwork quilt of lights spread beneath us and the moon's progress across the sky. Our short walk back to our hotel ended what would have been a perfect day, except for the emotional undercurrent of how important tomorrow was.

The next day brought the weather Seattle is famous for—cloudy skies and a mist of rain. Bob took the required Fleets enema and was still cramping when he came out of the bathroom. We dressed for cool weather, Bob in flannel slacks, striped shirt, subdued knit tie, and black wool blazer and me in a black wool pants-suit. Bob carried his umbrella; we anticipated needing it. Though it was past the rush hour at 9:30, the bellboy had trouble finding us a cab.

We arrived at a three-story brick building adjacent to Northwest Hospital and found Suite 106, a plain wooden door with a sign beside it that said: Haakon Ragde, F.A.C.S., Adult and Pediatric Urology. This introduced us to the low-keyed nature of the most famous urologist for seed implantation in the United States.

Dr. Ragde refined a technique developed by Dr. Hans Holms at the University of Copenhagen and brought it to Northwest Hospital in 1985. Dr. Ragde's team was the first in the U. S. to use ultrasound to guide placement of radioactive seeds into the prostate without open surgery. The Northwest Hospital team was also the first to use a computer to plan the radiation dose. These improvements allowed the seeds to be evenly spread throughout the prostate without damaging the nearby healthy tissue.

Dr. Ragde's jammed waiting room had no available seats. Bob leaned against a wall with his documents behind him on the floor, while he filled out the forms for a new patient. Dr. Ragde walked out of his office and saw Bob in that uncomfortable position. The doctor had no idea that Bob was a doctor, too. The message he'd left on our telephone was for Mr. Fine, because Bob's medical records read Robert A. Fine.

"You come into my office and fill those out," Dr. Ragde said.

Bob scooped up his documents and registration forms, and we walked into Dr. Ragde's office, the first on the left.

"Hi, I'm Doctor Bob Fine."

"I'm Saralee Fine."

He introduced himself, shook our hands, and walked out the door.

Bob filled out forms, while I looked around the tiny office. There was only one small window through which to monitor the gloomy day that matched our mood. Near it stood a computer and a light box with 35-mm. slides, probably exhibits included in the papers he wrote. Dr. Ragde's desk looked as if it had given him years of service. His chair appeared used and comfortable, too.

We sat on a couch longer than the width of his desk. Bob sat down first. An afterthought, the oversized sofa stood so close to the desk that Bob couldn't get out unless I moved first. Dr. Ragde's bookcases overflowed with books, medical journals, and papers. Snapshots of two horses, a grey and a dark flashy bay, leaned against them.

"Look at those photos, Bob," I said. "He's into horses. His horses look like Holy Smoke and Plenty when they were younger."

"A fellow horse fan, good." Having filled out the forms, he asked, "Do you think we should go back to the waiting room?"

"I haven't seen anyone pass by on the way in or out, so there won't be any seats in the waiting room," I said. "Do you want to stand?"

"No, but I think he might need his office."

Dr. Ragde came back. Stocky and sturdy, he stood about five-foot-ten. He wore green surgical scrubs and a white lab coat. His lion's mane of hair and bouncy stride in rubber-bottomed loafers belied his seventy years.

He sat at his desk, leaned back in his chair, stretched his arms, and put his hands behind his head. "What can I do for you?" he asked.

"Implant surgery," Bob said. "That's why I'm here."

Dr. Ragde nodded and smiled.

"Do you have your biopsy slides with you?"

"Yes."

"Are they labeled?"

"No, they're not. Maybe they don't label them in Atlanta."

"He didn't label them?"

"No, but I have my MRI with me, and the radiologists think . . . "

"MRI won't tell you much."

"Right."

"For instance, microscopic disease. Very few things pick up the microscopic stuff."

I shuddered inwardly. Now we were back at micro-metastases.

"Nothing actually, except the biopsy. Not the MRI," he said.

"Well, the radiologists think they saw something on the left side. Say, I thought we were supposed to meet at 1:15. But if you want to meet now instead, that's great."

He nodded. I guessed that he sensed how anxious we felt.

"Was the MRI done before or after the biopsy?" he asked.

"After."

"Yuh, then what they saw on the MRI may be blood left over from biopsy. Sometimes it can give a false positive, too."

"Yes."

"Well, there are three things you have to look at with treatment for prostate cancer. You know, how effective is the treatment, and right now we have actually—uh, I'm getting ready for ten-year data in another couple of months. January, I have 155 patients in ten years."

"That will be . . . "

"I just put together this morning an abstract for the AUA talking about observed rather than actuarial five-year data. These are patients I have seen, actual patients, over five years, 441 patients and looking at the PSA . . . . PSA is probably the best end-point we have."

His accent was fascinating, a mixture of Pacific Northwest and Scandinavian. His voice was animated, and his style of speech, informal.

"And at five years, we have a PSA equal to or less than 1. We have 83% in five years."

"And that is comparable to same stage surgery?"

"Yuh. It's comparable to Walsh's patients."

Walsh is Dr. Patrick Walsh, the urologic-surgery guru at Johns Hopkins in Baltimore.

"So it's just as good as the best surgical results actually in five years. And if you say, put PSA at 0.5, well, I don't buy it. Because as the prostate fibroses, you're going to get less and less PSA produced, so with time it will go down."

Fibrosis refers to tissues becoming scarred from the radiation from the implanted seeds. I hadn't realized that the seeds would scar Bob's prostate gland.

"But if you take this endpoint of 0.5, that's if you remove the prostate, it's 72%, so we're pretty close. These are the data we have. So I think right now, we have seven– and eight–year data, too, and seven– and eight–year data as good as the best possible surgery. Those are actuarial data. These are real. Real people."

"Yes, right."

'Now let me see if we have anything else here."

He looked through some papers, probably Bob's test results, and he hummed, the sound of a comfortable man.

"The second thing you look for is complications. The dreaded complications of prostate cancer. Incontinence is one. Impotence is another one. You are potent now?"

"Yes."

"Quite," I said.

"Yuh. Right. Good."

"But I have psychological overlay. When I turned sixty-five I had a problem."

"Well, a lot of people do."

"But that was purely psychological. Now it's all over."

"It's called menopause, male menopause," Dr. Ragde said, as he smiled at me.

"Is that what it was?" I said and giggled.

He had made me laugh for the first time that day.

"We have no incontinence with seeding if you haven't had previous surgery on your prostate."

"No, I haven't."

"With radical prostatectomy surgery, in good hands there is 20% incontinence. In bad hands, 100% incontinence. A lot of urologists say 2%, but that's dripping incontinence like a leaky faucet. But stress incontinence is very high. At least 20% in good hands and 100% in bad hands."

Dr. Ragde paused and shifted position in his chair.

"External beam radiation has not panned out to be that effective. In the old days, you could get away with anything, you know. No matter what you did, you felt the nodule disappear, and that was a good sign. But now we have PSA. I just reviewed a Swedish article for the *Journal of Cancer*. In five years, they had 65% PSA elevation and positive biopsy after external beam radiation. They probably didn't get enough radiation."

"Right."

"With seeding with iodine, you get approximately 11,000 to 12,000 external beams, rads, you know."

"In my case, what seeds would you use?"

"Palladium or iodine, you could use either one. I have a very good article on iodine."

"Right, I have it with me."

That was the article Bob had practically memorized. An article he had underlined, so that he could explain its relevance to me.

"August, *Cancer*," Dr. Ragde said.

Bob lifted the top article from his manila folder and showed it to Dr. Ragde.

"Yuh, that's the one. That's the one, yuh. So these are good data. I don't think palladium is any better. Whatever you want. Since you're from Atlanta, maybe you want to support your local industry, Theragenics," he quipped.

"Yes, I called them. I thought they produced Iodine-125. I was going to buy their stock."

"Theragenics. Their stuff was pretty good, you know. They went from $3 to almost $50."

"Right, but they do only palladium."

"North American Scientific is another company down in California. They went from $3 to $25 without producing a single seed, just on the come-on."

"Wow."

"That was about a month ago. I don't know what's happening now. I gave a talk at the Atomic Energy Commission, and I met somebody there, a fellow who is vice-president of a new company they have started in Texas called, let me see, International Isotopes. It's on the NASDAQ. It went public at $9, and I bought some at $10. They have the super-collider linear accelerator, you know."

I hadn't the foggiest notion what that was and guessed Bob didn't either. Talking stocks with Dr. Ragde made Bob feel at ease, as if he were comparing buys and sells with his Atlanta internist after an ordinary physical. Dr. Ragde had the knack of filing away the jagged edge of fear.

"That machine is very powerful. They can produce any type of isotope with it, and they can produce it faster and better than anyone else. They'll be in production within a year. I think that very few people know about this company."

"Uh huh."

"So if you're looking at . . . I wouldn't buy Theragenics now. I bought some of that new stuff after I had dinner with the vice president of International Isotopes."

Bob started laughing. Dr. Ragde's enthusiasm and candor delighted him.

"And they're going to just be wholesalers. They're not going to be retailers."

"I see. Well, there's such a demand."

"Right now, there sure is. So then we have impotence. How old are you now?"

"Sixty-five."

"Yuh, your age group, 20% impotency. With surgery, probably 70% to 100%. If you are very active sexually, your chance of impotency with seeds is probably much less than in your age group, too. Side effects of this thing is irritative and obstructive. And it's just temporary. Usually temporary. Rectal complication we usually don't have."

"Do you overload the periphery and underload around the urethra?"

"Yuh, we do a little, what we call, urethra-sparing. See, if you do it in dose volume histogram, you get a . . ."

He drew a sketch for us with two intersecting arcs.

"Here is the prostate sitting in here. And here is iodine, 16,000 rads, across this line here."

He was pointing out things to us as he talked, but they were incomprehensible to me.

"If you do uniform loading you get a dose that's something like this. Well, this is up to 30,000 rads. You don't really need that. If you do peripheral loading, it goes the other way round. So this is a more heterogeneous distribution. It turns out to be more homogeneous in the central part of the gland. What we do is something in between, probably."

"I see."

I hoped Bob did see and understand, because I didn't

"That we call urethral-sparing. We move the seeds a little away from the urethra. You still get a tremendous dose in there. Actually the normal urethra tolerates that dose, but if you have had TURP, you couldn't tolerate it too well."

"No."

TURP means trans-urethral resected prostate. It is a surgical procedure for men whose large prostate obstructs urination. The surgeon goes in through the urethra and removes a section of the prostate, so the man can urinate more easily.

"Actually, after seed implantation, the people I do go back to the hotel, maybe lie down for an hour, and then go out for dinner in Seattle."

"Great," Bob said.

Dr. Ragde made seeding sound easy and agreeable.

"Or go back to work the same day," Dr. Ragde continued.

"Does that mean we don't have to even stay over in Seattle for a few days?" I asked, incredulous with relief.

"Well, you have to stay overnight to have some dosimetry."

The dosimetry would consist of a CT scan and a chest X-ray to be certain the seeds had been properly placed and that none had strayed elsewhere.

"The next day?" Bob asked.

Dr. Ragde nodded and asked, "Do you have specific questions?"

"I guess I was going to ask would you use iodine in my case?"

"Well, whatever you want."

"No, that's up to you. You know much more than I do."

"Palladium would be over faster, but you ask Dr. Meier. Palladium is a little hard to get right now."

"Palladium is in Atlanta," I said and hoped some doctor in Atlanta could squirrel a dose of palladium for Bob from Theragenics.

"Tell Meier you want palladium, because you come from Atlanta," he said jovially.

"I was at Sloan Kettering," he continued. "Let me tell you a little bit about palladium. It has a low energy and travels very short distances. Actually, that's the reason we have so few complications, because outside the prostate you get very little radiation. Effective radiation is what, five millimeters around the prostate?"

"If you say so."

"With all this at Sloan Kettering, they did a model mathematical study using carcinoma of the tongue. That's a totally different cancer from that of the prostate. I'm not sure you can extrapolate between the two. The conclusion was that iodine was better for slow-growing tumors and palladium was better for fast-growing tumors."

"Yes, that's what I found in my reading, too."

"Well, what they call a rapidly growing tumor, you know. In the prostate, most of them are slow-growing."

"Yes."

"So whatever. But it has never been tested clinically."

"But the Iodine-125 has been used a lot more, is that right?"

"Well, yuh. This paper I just did now, I had, uh . . . See, Palladium-103 did not become available until 1987. I put the first palladium seed in right here. 345 patients treated with iodine and 98 with palladium; ⅓ of the patients got palladium, because it's a later isotope. Actually one of the advantages of palladium is that it's over faster. You recover faster."

"I see."

"All the side effects, urethral, rectal, are over in six months."

"So you prefer the palladium," I said.

"I don't prefer anything. I like both of them. Do you know Dr. Shipley at Harvard?"

"No."

"He's one of the big-time radiation oncologists, and he got a bit upset with me. I was on a committee with him, and he likes external beam. I countered him pretty heavily. He had rented a car. He wanted somebody to travel around with him, so I traveled around with him. He kept telling me to cool it on this iodine, because he could guarantee me iodine was no good. Because he had done some work on it in England in the early days."

"Was he right?"

"As soon as I got back, I did my iodine study, and I was surprised myself how good it was."

"Excellent."

"I was at Sloan Kettering in the '60's when we did the early implants."

"The seed placement was inaccurate then," Bob said.

"We selected our patients. We had a terrible selection of patients. We thought we could seed anybody. As long as the prostate was free, as long as you could move the gland away from the pelvis. So these people were not candidates to be cured for anything. Number one, we didn't have PSA. Number two, we did open dosimetry."

Open dosimetry implies random seed placement.

"We had a carpenter's measurement. Up there in the operating room, we measured the length, width, and height. Estimated the height usually. And then we did a graphic type of dosimetry. And now we know that it was very wrong. And then we put the seeds in free-hand, and usually we got more heterogeneity than homogeneity of placement.

"We had a poor selection of patients, poor dosimetry, and poor placement of seeds. Neither iodine nor palladium could be effective under these circumstances."

"I have a question," I said. "I have lupus, so exposure to radiation is a bad thing for me. After this procedure is done, can we sleep in the same bed?"

"Sure, no problem."

"Can I hug him?"

"Sure. You get very little radiation out front here. Matter of fact, you can put a child on your lap for three hours on the airplane and fly to Denver. The child will get about one millirad of radiation. Behind, you get more radiation, in front of the rectum. But nobody's going to sit on you there, except a chair."

We both laughed at his geniality. He made treating Bob's cancer and the effects afterward seem simple.

"So there's very little radiation outside the prostate."

"Now," Bob said, "You're doing most of these with Dr. Meier?"

"I train all the radiologic oncologists and work with them—Meier, Blasko. I was the one who learned how to do it and brought it here."

"I know," Bob said. "And then Blasko left. I've heard about that."

"It happens, you know."

"For sure," I said and remembered Bob's unsavory split from his partners ten years ago.

"But Blasko hadn't done one implant. I do all the implants, over 2,000 of them. Though he worked with me on dosimetry and everything like that."

"You as the urologist are the most essential," Bob said.

"I do all the implants."

"When would you be able to do this for Bob?" I asked softly.

This was the essential question. When could Bob's cancer be treated? When could we stop worrying? How soon?

"What?"

I repeated the question in a louder voice.

"See when Dr. Meier can fit you in. We'll try to do this as soon as we can. When he can get palladium. Right now, I get phone calls every day to go places, to give talks."

"Right," Bob said.

"And I try to do half of them, maybe."

"Can you put me at ease by assuring me that if I have to wait four or six or maybe even ten weeks for palladium that nothing's going to progress?"

"Well, it's not going to happen. See what Meier will do. Tell him that I suggested he get you in earlier."

"Okay. All right. Thank you."

"Matter of fact it's not necessary that you use palladium. I always use it with Gleason 7 to 10, because those are more virulent cancers. You have a Gleason 6, so either Palladium-103 or Iodine-125 would do. Palladium is hard to find quickly. Talk to Meier."

"Yes, I will."

"This is an article that, without my knowledge, appeared in *The London Times*. He was from the BBC, pretty well known guy. Humphrey Burton. He goes up to Tanglewood and directs music there. He wrote the biography of Leonard Bernstein, a book this thick."

He spread his thumb and a finger to three or four inches.

"Thank you."

Dr. Ragde left his office.

"It sounds as if he'd like to use palladium," I whispered to Bob.

"He would favor it, but that's not up to him. He won't make that decision. It's the radiologist who will make the decision."

"I see. It can't be such a horrible procedure, after all. Guys go out for dinner that night," I said and smiled.

"Right-o," Bob said, up-beat.

"What we need now are available seeds."

"Well, Meier, the radiologist here at this center, would have more influence than anybody. If he will make that phone call."

"I hope he'll do that for us."

"I'm a little surprised by the fact that Dr. Ragde doesn't favor palladium strongly over iodine. He said that radiation from palladium is more intense and that the half-life of the material is shorter."

I would learn by reading a booklet written for Northwest Hospital and called "Seeds of Hope, Seeds of Health" that the half-life of palladium is seventeen days and that of iodine, sixty days. Half-life is the number of days it takes for half the radiation to dissipate. For example, in sixty days half of the Iodine-125 radiation is gone. In another sixty days, half the remaining radiation is gone, and so on.

The radiation of palladium decays in six months. It takes twelve months for iodine to become inactive, so the process of recovery takes twice as long. Still, iodine had the longer track record. The inactive seeds would remain in Bob's prostate without any reactions.

Our interview seemed finished, so we wandered out of Dr. Ragde's office and into the waiting room where we found chairs which were not together. I talked with a young woman who lived in Seattle. Her father had been treated by Dr. Ragde with hormones, exterior beam radiation, and seed implantation.

"When my parents come to Seattle to see Dr. Ragde, I'm the hotel," she said. "Dad was such an active man before this. The treatment really drained him, but he's doing better now."

Dr. Ragde came to summon his next patient. I thought it quaint that this famous urologist calls his patients in personally rather than using his secretary. A wife accompanied that patient, so Bob and I sat together. I put my arm alongside his, reassured by his touch.

"Look at that man," he said and pointed at someone in a plaid shirt and a green sweater. "He sounds like a Southerner. I'll bet they're from the South, just like us."

We sat quietly together until a secretary called Bob's name and led us to the room where a volume survey would be done.

BOB

The ultrasound technician talked a mile a minute. The first thing he said was surprising and reassuring. That young man had done over 8,000 ultrasound exams of the prostate. I was glad such an experienced tech had chosen to stay with Ragde instead of going with Blasko.

I hoped the physicist had stayed here, too. He was an important member of the team, because his mathematical skills would help Dr. Meier plan my treatment.

"I'll get you out of here in fifteen minutes, while others would take an hour to do the same procedure," the tech said.

That sounded like egotistical exaggeration.

"I'm good, and I'm fast. Look at my schedule for today."

I looked at the long schedule taped to his door, one study every twenty or thirty minutes. I felt like part of his production line. He seemed both excited and perturbed by his schedule, hyped up.

"I'm Dr. Bob Fine," I said, "a radiologist."

I told him that, hoping he would slow his pace and take better care of me. I took off my blazer, belt, slacks, underwear, and shoes. I nervously undid my tie and opened my shirt collar.

"No, you don't need your shirt and tie off. Come on."

I climbed onto his examining table and put my feet in the stirrups. I kept telling myself to relax. His attitude had made me uptight, and that had tightened my anal sphincter.

His lubricating gel felt cold on my anus. Rapidly, he slid a lubricated ultrasound probe with a balloon at its end into place high in my rectum. He inflated the balloon.

"How are you tolerating this?" he asked.

"It's uncomfortable, but I can tolerate it. Have you ever done this on a patient who liked it?" I said and hoped to befriend him with a joke.

"Nope, and if he liked it, I'd get out of the room fast."

While he was doing the examination, I could watch my ultrasound on a screen that he had facing me. It seemed weird to see a projection of myself on that screen. My prostate was inert, impersonal. I wished that it weren't mine.

The technician would move the probe, freeze the position, and rush the few feet to a stool beside another screen where he'd outline my prostate gland and print an image. I kept trying to see the tumor.

"Do you see the tumor?" I asked.

"Maybe in the apex."

He kept outlining, drawing lines, getting the contour and volume on multiple images. I felt as if my prostate and I myself were being put to the test. What if the cancer had spread out of the gland capsule, and this trip to Seattle were wasted? I thought, please don't let this happen to me.

"Yes, your gland is enlarged," he said. "Let's keep taking measurements."

I feared that my enlarged gland was proof that this trip had been made in vain. I wouldn't be allowed to have the treatment I wanted.

"We'll have to measure your pubic arch," he said.

Here was yet another reason to reject me as a seeding candidate. I doubted that he could study my pubic arch with ultrasound.

"I have small bones," I said.

I wondered if he were referring to the angle of my arch instead of my bone size.

I felt glad that I'd never had a fracture there, or I certainly couldn't have the seed implants. Until this ultrasound, I had felt certain both my prostate gland and pubic arch were acceptable for radioactive seeding. Now this tech had filled me with doubts. He jinxed me.

The technician kept talking and talking. He'd say, 'In my humble opinion' this and 'In my humble opinion' that as if he wanted me to respond, "You're not humble, and your opinions are brilliant."

Then he began overstepping his bounds, extending his role. He talked about implanting extra seeds here, implanting extra seeds there. My ultrasound tech chats too much with patients. But this tech was impossible, a non-stop talker who knew all the wrong things to say.

Dr. Ragde came into the examining room. I didn't know why he was there. Maybe something had gone wrong with my exam. Maybe he was just checking on me, another caretaking gesture. The tech shut up as long as my doctor stayed in the room.

When the tech had finished the exam and removed the probe, he rushed out of the room with images of my prostate printed on paper. I assumed he would turn them over to Dr. Ragde.

He turned at the door, put a finger near his lips, and said, "Not a word of what I've told you to anyone."

Of course. Because he had no authority to say most of those things. I was glad to see him go. I cleaned up the lubricant as best I could with a box of tissues he'd handed me. I did not change my underpants, though we had brought an extra pair with us. Perhaps I'd have diarrhea later from the enema that morning. I finished dressing. We were leaving when the tech rushed back into the room.

"Your pubic arch looks good," he said "You're all set."

I liked him for that good news and forgave his constant chattering.

"Wait," he said. "I want to show you something I'm working on."

It was a schematic on his computer. A red prostate gland had multiple needles, sleeves filled with radioactive seeds, embedded into and protruding from it. The technician could rotate the gland on his screen to show the implant procedure from all angles. I was fascinated.

"Dr. Ragde wants to see you before you go," he said.

Saralee and I walked to down the hall to Dr. Ragde's office, and he met us at the door.

"Everything has gone well this morning. You are officially a candidate for brachytherapy."

Brachytheraphy is the scientific term for radioactive seed implantation.

"Great," I said and smiled with gratitude and relief.

"We think the tumor is on the right side, not the left. That's unimportant. When I've finished seeding you, your entire prostate will begin dying."

"That's exactly what I want."

"It doesn't matter whether I use palladium or iodine. Get with Meier and see what he says. I'll do what I can to match my schedule with available seeds. I'll work you in."

My hunger announced noon. We stopped at a snack bar in the building.

"Where's a good place to eat?"

The lady behind the counter seemed nonplused and said, "There's a Barnaby's in a shopping center nearby. It's pretty good."

"Is there anywhere to eat at the hospital?" I asked and pointed to Northwest Hospital, the next building.

"Sure," she said. "There's a coffee shop there."

It was drizzling lightly as we walked to the hospital, not enough to need my umbrella. Just enough to make the grey day hazier. Inside I gravitated toward a coffee shop on the left.

"Wait a minute," Saralee said. "We're at a major medical center. The staff must have a place for meals. I'll bet outpatients can eat there, too."

She went to a "pink" lady behind a desk who directed us to the hospital cafeteria with endless food choices. Now I felt more tired than hungry, so I chose only soup and a salad. Saralee said she wasn't hungry at all; she rarely eats lunch.

She eyed my vegetable soup and said, "Yummers."

"Go get a bowl and a spoon. I'll share it with you."

She came back with a plastic spoon and a styrofoam cup. I put a couple of spoonfuls into the cup, and she ate the soup.

"This tastes terrific, the perfect medicine for a cold on a mucky day," she said.

"Go get a bowl for yourself."

She did and found a slice of blackberry pie that I couldn't resist.

"Ragde never seemed rushed this morning, though his office was filled with patients," I said.

"He was incredibly generous to us."

"Busy as can be, yet he never seemed hassled."

"He's a special breed of doctor who puts you at ease."

"He really cares."

It was only slightly past noon when we finished eating, and our appointment with Dr. Robert Meier wasn't until two o'clock. As we had nothing better to do, we followed the directions Dr. Ragde's secretary had given us to Dr. Meier's office. We would read in his waiting room until my appointment. Maybe Dr. Meier would see us early, as Dr. Ragde had.

I went to the desk, told them my name, and asked for the registration forms I'd certainly need to fill out.

"You're not due here until two," a receptionist said. "Why not go and eat lunch?"

"I've already done that. If you give me the necessary forms, I'll fill them out. Then we'll sit in a corner of the waiting room until Dr. Meier can see me."

It was a very large waiting room and almost empty except for the patients being wheeled in and out for therapy at the tumor clinic adjacent to the therapeutic-radiology department.

We tried to read, but I had trouble concentrating on *The New Yorker,* and Saralee was turning few pages in her book. We sat beside one another, twin bumps on a log. We wished the next appointment were over, wished the seeds had been ordered, wished the implant had been done.

I saw a man with Dr. Robert something sewn on his lab coat pocket and assumed he was my doctor on his way to lunch. I saw him return some time later. My name was called at two o'clock, and a woman led us to an examining room.

"Hello," she said, "I'm Dr. Meier's nurse. It's been a good day for me. I've just found a dose of Palladium-103 for a lucky man by the end of December."

"That's more than two months from now," I said.

"The waiting time for palladium is well over three months. The wait time for iodine is shorter."

She took my blood pressure.

"It's elevated," she said.

"Yours would be, too, if you felt like I do: worried, tense, worked up."

"I'm sorry. We're going to help you. You'll see," she said and left the room.

I turned to Saralee and said, "Oh, brother. I want this over with sooner than three months from now."

As answer, she shrugged.

Dr. Meier arrived. He was younger than both Dr. Ragde and I. He had nicely greying sideburns and a thick head of hair. His dark eyes seemed friendly and caring. He smiled as we all introduced our-selves.

Dr. Meier asked me to tell him about the rectal ultrasound that was done in Atlanta.

"My urologist did the digital. I asked him if he felt any nodules, and he said, 'No.' Then, he did the ultrasound. I asked, 'Is there any-thing suspicious?' and he said, 'No, no. Well maybe.'"

"He biopsied your prostate, didn't he?"

"Yes, he did six quadrant cores. He said, 'While you're here, lets play it safe and do them.' So he did the biopsy. When we met later, he said, 'There's a millimeter focus of malignancy in one of the six cores.'"

"Yes, okay."

"And you may not have a copy of Jonathan Epstein's report, but he agreed it was a Gleason 6."

"You've got it with you?"

"Yes."

I handed the report to Dr. Meier. I had found it while we sat in the waiting room, when I opened the two packets of biopsy slides to combine them. One held the three slides that Johns Hopkins in Baltimore had promptly sent back to Atlanta. The other held the six slides Johns Hopkins had misplaced and sent later. Dr. Epstein's report was with those six.

"Good, they're graded. That's because Epstein does a lot of them. I want a copy of this."

"All right."

He went out to make a copy.

"What do you think of him?" I asked Saralee.

"He seems okay. I wish he'd get to the bottom line, like when can he get the seeds."

"Be patient. He needs to go through his routine. To cover what he's going to do in his own way."

Dr. Meier returned and handed me the report. If Saralee thought me hyper-reactive for having my slides read by several pathologists at two Atlanta hospitals and then sending them on to Epstein, she ought to feel differently now. Even though my slides had been lost twice along the way, Dr. Epstein's report was specific and necessary.

"All right," Dr. Meier said, "have you had any other diagnostic studies?"

"I had an MRI. It showed no spread out of the gland."

"I saw that."

"I had an acid phosphatase within normal limits."

"I saw that."

"And no bone scan. The urologist said it was a waste of time."

"I think he's right. The odds of having it spread to the bones with a PSA of less than 4 is minuscule. It's not cost effective to do the procedure. But if you want one for the sake of easing anxiety, I'll order it."

"No, I don't need one. The urologist thought the acid phosphatase and the MRI were a waste of time, too."

"The MRI is easily misinterpreted. It can be a red herring. Any other symptoms, any other changes recently?"

I liked Dr. Meier. He was thorough. I could talk to him easily. I told him about my emotional hit at turning sixty-five, my high blood pressure and its medication, and my impotence, all of which had cleared.

"So you can attain an erection sufficient to have intercourse."

"Yes."

"Beautifully," Saralee said.

"You've got a witness," he said and laughed. "That's important as you know. Because the treatment for prostate cancer can affect sexual potency. Have you ever had a transurethral resection of the prostate?"

"No, no," I said emphatically.

"The reason I ask that is because it changes the complication rate with this procedure, and we might do things a little bit differently. Have you discussed treatment options with Dr. Ragde?"

"Oh, yes," I said. "Before I came here, I did months of reading. I've talked to a lot of doctors. I've talked to a lot of patients. Yes, I'm quite aware of the options."

"Good. You've educated yourself."

"Yes. Since I believe that the cancer is confined to the gland, there should be fewer complications with implantation. I've come to the conclusion that seeds are what's best for me."

"Okay, we'll talk more about that. Even though I know you're informed, I'd like to make sure I've explained things."

I understood that he had a path that he normally followed with a new patient, and that he would waltz me down it despite what I knew. I admired him for that.

"Who is your urologist in Atlanta?"

"He's," I said, then paused. I felt tired.

Saralee gave him his name and added, "He's a urologist and an oncologist. Both specialties."

"Oh," Dr. Meier said. "I need to examine you, if you don't mind."

"I won't say, 'my pleasure.' But yes," I said.

"I'll examine your heart and lungs first. I'll just ask you to take off your tie and shirt, if you don't mind."

"Sure."

"I can get you a gown."

"I don't need it."

"You're okay? All right."

He examined my heart and lungs.

"Dr. Ragde said, after my ultrasound had been done, he was thinking of treating the whole gland equally, as if there were tumor throughout. Not that there is. Not to localize it to one area."

"We always do that. In every patient we treat, we do the whole gland. The reason for that is . . . . It's a little bit like what the surgeon does. The surgeon doesn't just remove the cancer in one area."

"Right."

"Oftentimes, there will be more disease than we see on biopsy, and the ultrasound is really not too specific for showing us where tumor is. We have to treat the whole gland. That's standard procedure. You haven't noticed any swollen lymph nodes, have you?"

"No, I check my groin."

He checked it, too, and the nodes on my neck.

"I'm just checking everything I can."

"You know, I'm almost blind in one eye and have been since birth," I said for completeness and felt that I could level with him.

He thumped on my back to see if it hurt.

"Nobody in your family has had prostate cancer?"

"No"

"That's good. It does increase the risk for cancer if a family member's had it."

He put a glove on his right hand and said, "I have to, uh . . . "

"I understand. Do you want me on my right side or left side?"

"Maybe if you just stand up and turn around."

"Now don't look," I said to Saralee.

"Do you mind if your wife stays in the room?"

"I don't mind. She's seen me naked many times before."

"Drop your pants and underpants. Lean over right here."

"Right here"meant the end of the examining table.

"A little farther. All right."

I did as told. He used lots of lubricant and kept poking around up my rectum. I hoped it was the last time today that my ass-hole would be assaulted.

You can't clear your rectum of all that lube. There was some in my underpants already, and now there would be more. No matter how carefully I cleaned myself up.

Still I didn't want to change into clean underpants, for fear I could have loose stools from the enema. I did have more diarrhea. But that was later, when we were safely back at our hotel.

"Oh, your prostate is large," he sighed compassionately.

When he had finished examining me, he said, "I don't feel anything. No nodules."

"Great."

"You can use that to wipe yourself off," he said and handed me the obligatory box of tissues.

He removed his glove and washed his hands, while I did what I could for myself. I'm sure he was a lot cleaner than I when we had both finished.

"Did Dr. Ragde say this was approachable without any prostate shrinking?" he asked.

"Yes, that's what he told me."

"Your prostate is large. But not so large that we'll get pubic arch interference."

"That's what the ultrasoundographer said, too."

"All right. If you don't mind, I'll give you a little bit of my 'spiel.' But I'll cut it short, because I know that you know about it. So I'll cut everything short."

"Sure."

"Then we can talk about seed implants. You're sixty-five. Is that right?"

"Yes."

"As you know, when men get older, many of them get prostate cancer. If you look carefully at autopsies of men who die in their seventies and eighties of unrelated causes, over half of them have some prostate cancer."

"I've read that."

"Yet most of them had no idea they had it. So you can have prostate cancer, and it won't be a problem. In some people, as you know, prostate cancer can be a big problem. It can spread through the body and be fatal."

"Yes."

"We decide who to treat and who not to treat, because we don't want to treat all those people who have indolent disease."

Indolent disease is a tumor that is not causing any harm and is not expected to cause any harm.

"A couple of things are very important. One is the age of the person. If a person is older and has major medical problems, we don't need to treat it, because probably the cancer will never impact.

"If you're only sixty-five years of age, you need to think hard about having treatment. Because you stand to live twenty more years easily. And who knows what this cancer will do in twenty years. But I think you should be aware of the option of observation."

"Yes," I said softly, because I knew that observation alone would drive me crazy.

"Since you're here, I expect seed implantation is what you want."

"Unequivocally."

"Okay. Let's talk about the potential cure for treatment. Now the reason I say potential is that the cancer has to be limited to the gland. We think your cancer is limited to the gland, but our best diagnostic studies cannot predict microscopic disease elsewhere.

"So, there's a chance you can have disease that has spread through the blood already, but it's small. That's because your PSA is so low. The report of PSA results is an excellent indicator of success. Those with a PSA below 4 have the very best chance. Those between 4 and 10 have a good chance, too. When you get to 10 to 20, the number starts falling, because those patients have disease that has gotten into the blood stream and cannot be cured. So you are potentially curable."

"Curable. That's wonderful."

"The other thing to look at is a Gleason score. Do you know how a Gleason score works?"

"Yes."

"A lot of this is superfluous for you, and I apologize. I'm used to going through all the information."

"I know, and that's okay. I'm always learning."

He explained that a Gleason of 2 through 4 indicated only indolent disease, that 5 and 6 were intermediate, and that 7 through 10 were aggressive and hard to treat.

"Fortunately, you have a Gleason of 6; 3 and 3, and that's good," he said. "There's not much chance that this has spread to the lymph nodes or beyond that. So, you have a couple of good things to look at, your PSA and your Gleason. Your Gleason is intermediate, but given the PSA, I think it's a good combination."

"Good."

"On the other hand, there's the clinical findings. Yours is a T1c, which means we can't feel it. It was detected on an elevated PSA."

"T1a's and T1c's, are they clinically comparable?"

"No, T1c's are probably a little worse."

Saralee squirmed in her chair. She probably wished I'd stop asking questions. Even she knew the answer to that one.

"T1b's do a little worse than T1c's. That's probably what you're thinking about."

"Yes. Okay."

"T1a's are not usually treated. Some people treat them. Patrick Walsh does, but most people do not.

"Okay, that's the prognostic factors," Dr. Meier continued, "and I think you're in a good group. Now, where the treatment is concerned, there's radical surgery and there's radiation therapy. There are different ways of giving radiation therapy. I think you know about radical surgery, the pros and cons and the associated side effects."

Saralee was becoming restless. I wanted to touch her and assure her that he had to cover his groundwork, but she sat on a chair against the wall, and I was sitting on the edge of the examining table in the center of the room.

"In a young person who is still sexually active, impotence is a big deal. The likelihood of losing your ability to sustain an erection with radical surgery is close to 100%. In the nerve-sparing prostatectomy, it's less. It's anywhere between 30% to 70%, but it's unclear if the nerve-sparing procedure is as good as the radical procedure."

"Yes, I've been told that."

He explained external beam radiation and internal radiation.

"The internal radiation is why I'm here."

"There are two ways of doing it. There's seeding, which we do here and which a number of institutions are doing. There's also something they call a high-dose rate. That's where the needles are put into you. You're connected to a machine, and you stay in the hospital for a day or two. The sources come in and go out. That's another way of doing brachytherapy."

"There was an excellent article written by the CEO of Intel, Andy Grove. That's the therapy he had with a Gleason of 7 and a PSA of 6. You know, I've read that article many times. And he had these 'in and out' things done."

"My partner downtown did him. He came here. It's funny that

he went to two doctors from the same group. Doctors who work together.

"Now, the advantage of brachytherapy is that you get a high dose to the gland and very little to the surrounding tissues. We're limited in external radiation as to what we can give, because you have to treat through the bladder and the rectum. We can only give about 7,000 rads.

"Now, you can do conformal radiation with special techniques, and you can escalate the dose a little bit. But even then you can't safely do more than 7,500 rads."

"When does one do seeds and external radiation?"

"Excellent question. Most people don't even know that's an important issue. When there's a high likelihood of extracapsular disease."

Extracapsular disease refers to cancer that has spread outside of the prostate capsule.

"How do we know? We look at the literature of people who have had radical prostatectomy. What do they find? We find there's a high likelihood of that if the PSA is above 10 or the Gleason score is 7 or above, or if it's a high clinical score like a T2b and above. And sometimes combinations of those or slightly lower combinations will decide it."

"So that's not even a consideration in my case?"

"We have not treated people in your category with Gleason 6's and T1c's this way. It could be done. But our results are so good doing seeds alone. I don't think you need it."

"Okay. I just needed to get that off my mind."

"The advantage of doing the seeds is that we can give a high dose to one area. The bladder and rectal complications are less than if you give external beam. And the dose is higher to the prostate cancer, so we believe the control rates are higher.

"The side effects of this treatment are mostly to the urethra, also a little bit to the bladder, but mostly to the urethra. You have to get a high dose to the prostatic urethra. We'll talk about that. Maybe I can tell you about how the procedure works. Or do you know?"

"What I know is that they have a template, and they insert the sleeves with the seeds in them, then they take the sleeves out, and the radioactive seeds remain. It's done under spinal, and it should take less than an hour for the whole procedure."

"That's right. We use an ultrasound probe in the rectum, so we know exactly where we're putting them. There are generally about 25 to 30 needles and 80 to 100 seeds."

"Wow. That's a lot of needles and seeds. Dr Ragde has done over 2,000 cases. Will he be the man who inserts the seeds?"

"Yes. The urologist places the needles according to the plan we come up with."

"Who comes up with the plan, you and the physicist?"

"Yes. The plans are all fairly similar. There are only so many con-figurations of the prostate. The physicist comes up with a plan, and we tweak it a bit. Since you know how this works, let me tell you a little about the side effects of it."

"Okay."

"The acute side effects are from puncturing the skin of the per-ineum. You could get a hematoma, but probably not. You will get bruising which sometimes gravitates to the scrotum and penis. That gets better in a couple of days.

"After three or four days, you start to have some side effects from the radiation that is given off by the seeds. A patient develops uri-nary frequency, urgency, sometimes a burning when they urinate.

"Most patients get a decreased urinary stream. This peaks in one to two weeks, and then it gradually goes away over a period of weeks to months. Sometimes, it takes six to nine months for the flow to return to normal, but not usually. We'll give you medicines to help the flow."

He named the medications.

"Do any of these have side effects of impotence?"

"The Cardura, an alpha blocker can potentially have that effect, but it's transient for that month.

"Those side effects are right after treatment. There are others you live with for the rest of your like. So, if you don't mind, may I tell you about those?"

"Sure."

"Some patients will have a permanently decreased urinary stream. Maybe 5% to 10% will notice their stream is not as good, but only 1% or 2% have a stricture that requires a procedure to open it up."

A stricture is a narrowing of the urethra. The procedure would be to put a dilator up the urethra to widen it and break possible adhesions due to scar tissue formation.

"Incontinence is rare. If you haven't had a TURP, it's less than 1%. There's probably a 5% to 7% chance of having cystitis-like symptoms, inflammation of the bladder or urethra.

"What that means is there's a slight chance you'll have a change in your urinary habits. You may have to urinate more frequently or experience more urgency. You could have increased nocturnal urination, some of which you have now."

"Yes."

"Sexual function depends on the age of the patient and how they're doing to start with. With patients over seventy who are already having some difficulty getting an erection, over half will lose their ability to have an erection in five to eight years.

"If you take younger men who don't have a problem getting an erection, it's probably less—15% to 20% of them wind up in five to eight years losing their ability to have an erection. Now there might be some people, maybe 20% or 25%, who, over the next five to eight years, find their erection is not as good as it was. Probably what happens is that the radiation accelerates the natural process."

"Yes."

"Rectal symptoms and complications are uncommon. An ulceration of the rectum can happen, but it's rare, probably less than 1%. And there is probably a couple percent chance that you'll have some painless bleeding down the road, months to years later. If that happens, have it worked up, because it could be from other problems."

"Yes, I'd certainly do that."

"If someone looked into your rectum, they'd see some changes from the radiation where it's right up against the prostate."

"Oh, I didn't know that."

"It's possible to cause another cancer. Radiation can cause other cancers, but it takes a long time for another cancer to develop. I think that, given the delay in causing another malignancy, the risk that this cancer poses is much greater."

"I agree."

"Did I cover everything? I think so."

"How often after surgery does one have to be catheterized to be able to void, like the first day or second day?"

"That's a good question. I did miss something. Probably 10% of the patients have a catheter temporarily, for a few days or a few weeks. Those patients likely had obstructive symptoms to begin with. You don't have that. So I think it's unlikely that would happen, but it's possible."

I explained that Saralee had lupus and asked if we could sleep in the same bed after surgery.

Dr. Meier turned to Saralee and said, "You can sleep next to him. You can do anything you want."

"Great," she said.

"We are cautious, though. You should stand a few feet away from pregnant women and not have infants or small children sit on your lap for long periods of time for six months afterwards."

"All right. I prefer the surgery done in the morning. Everybody's fresh then."

"Okay."

"So let's say it's done in the morning. I would stay overnight in Seattle. When would we be able to fly home to Atlanta?"

"Late the following day. You come in a day before the procedure, so we can do a little bowel prep. We don't want stool there. Then we do the surgery the next day. The day after the procedure we need to do a CT scan of the area where we put the seeds. We need to do that for our quality assurance reasons. Then you can leave."

"When you do the CT scan, if you see seeds out of place, I know you can't take them out. Do you ever add any seeds?" I asked.

"We haven't had to add any. There's been a couple of cases where we've given external beam radiation to one spot."

"How often does that happen?"

"I think it's happened two or three times out of 2,000 or 3,000 cases. It's pretty unlikely."

"I just need to plan for everything."

"If the CT scan taken the day after surgery could be done early in the morning, we would take the noon flight to Atlanta," Saralee said. "Otherwise we'd have to be on the red eye, and we're both too old for that."

"Everybody hates the red eye anyhow," Dr. Meier said and chuckled.

"How much pain will Bob be in? We usually fly economy, because both ends of the plane land at the same time. Will we need to travel back first class?"

"I think you'll be okay. You'll have a little discomfort, but you'll be okay."

"Dr. Ragde said Bob could go out for dinner that night."

"Yes. I know some people who play golf the next day."

"Do I have to stay away from any physical activity like lifting?"

"We ask people not to exert themselves heavily for the first two weeks, so the seeds don't come out. I'm not sure it makes a difference."

"All right."

"If you have intercourse within two weeks afterwards, you may have some discomfort from the procedure and also with ejaculation. You should wear a condom, because occasionally a seed will come out in the semen. You don't want to deposit it in your partner. We also get a chest X-ray, because occasionally a seed will become an embolus and travel to your lungs. It doesn't do anything."

"Just good to know about it."

"That's a lot of information I've given you."

"Is there any extra benefit using the Iodine-125 or the Palladium-103?"

"We don't know, because we haven't compared the data. We should do that study. We usually use iodine with a Gleason of 6 or below and palladium on 7 and above. But sometimes we use them with Gleason 6. You could do either one. It makes no difference."

"Okay."

"I would use iodine. It can be gotten quicker."

"How quickly can it be gotten?" Saralee said in a quiet voice, the serious voice she uses to say 'please' when she's dependent on someone to get her out of a bind.

"Yes, can you push it?" I continued. "I want to get it done fast."

"Yes."

"Dr. Ragde said he could do this anytime," Saralee said. "He'll be in and out of town, but he can do it anytime."

"Let me get the book."

"Okay, great," I said and began feeling hopeful.

"Be back in a minute."

"Moving along," I said to him.

He left and I said, "Oh, am I tired! He went through everything. He was so thorough. I appreciated that."

"Yes. He was too thorough."

"That's his routine. Also, for medical legal reasons, he did it."

"Oh," she said, surprised. "I never thought of that."

"May I?" I asked and reached for her hand.

"Certainly, and I'm stroking back."

SARALEE

We sat close together until Dr Meier returned with his schedule book.

"Your studies will be complete and your seeds can be here by November 11th. I can do you then, but it won't be in the morning," Dr. Meier said. "It will be at 1:45."

"That's okay," Bob said. "November 11th is only three-and-a-half weeks from now."

"Let me go out and check the time with Dr. Ragde's office."

"I'm elated," Bob said.

"Me, too," I said.

"It'll be all over in less than four weeks."

"Sorry," Dr. Meier said as he walked in. "Dr. Ragde can't do it until November 25th. He'll be away giving symposiums for other doctors, training them in seed-implantation techniques."

"But he said he'd be in and out of town. And promised he'd get this done as soon as you could get seeds."

"Yes."

"We're both so troubled. Bob wants this over with."

"Preferably yesterday," Bob said.

"I understand," Dr. Meier said. "If it were me, I'd want the same. I can do it any Tuesday after November 11th, whenever Dr. Ragde wants."

Tuesday was the day for seed implantations.

"Let's go back upstairs to Dr. Ragde's office and see what we can work out," I said.

We walked up the flight of stairs and talked with his secretary. She told us he wouldn't be available until November 25th. We asked to see him, and she complied.

"Dr. Ragde," Bob said, "I'm so tense and worried with this thing growing inside me. What can you do to help?"

"I'll put you on Proscar, 5 mg. and Casodex, 50 mg. per day."

He wrote the names of the drugs on a sheet from his legal pad and handed it to Bob.

"You can write your own prescriptions in Georgia, right?"

"Right, but what will they do?"

"They'll make your prostate even more receptive to the radiation. Will you take those medicines, please?"

"If you really think I need them," Bob said reluctantly.

I was skeptical. If Dr. Ragde truly thought Bob needed those medications, he'd have said so that morning.

"What are the side effects?" I asked.

"Every medication has side effects," he answered.

"That's why I'm asking."

"Among other things, it lowers the libido."

I made a sour face.

"It's only for five or six weeks. The man says he's worried."

I made another sour face and said, "Not worried enough to ruin our sex life."

"Perhaps you would like my associate, Dr. Kenny, to do the surgery. He can do it sooner."

"We came all the way to Seattle for you to be his surgeon."

"I'm sorry. I'm so busy."

He got a book out of his pocket. It was his calendar.

"I leave for Belgium next week. Then I go to Pittsburgh to teach and give a symposium. I'm back here November 3rd and 4th. Then I'm away until November 24th."

I had taken my calendar out of my purse.

"November 4th is a Tuesday. Could you do it then?"

"Yes, if Meier can get the seeds."

He called Meier's office, and they talked. He had his secretary bring his schedule book.

"You're already booked for that day," she said.

"I can do ten a day; we have six scheduled."

He looked at Bob and said, "I can do you on November 4th at 10:15 A.M. That's less than three weeks from now. Okay?"

"It's more than okay, it's spectacular," Bob said.

He stood, and we, also.

"I could hug you," Bob said.

"Me, too." I said, but we were too much in awe of him to do that.

We stopped at the reception desk where we received requests for an EKG and a blood work-up.

"Do you want them done here or when you get home?" the receptionist asked.

"I might as well have them done here. That way, they can't get lost."

"We also need the report from a current chest X-ray."

"I'll send you that. It was taken at my hospital, and I interpreted the films myself."

As we opened the door, Dr. Meier was standing outside. He had come to meet us.

"Come down to my office," he said.

He began explaining on the way down, "We do so many seed implants here that we place an order for what we need each Friday. We've already faxed Nycomed Amersham today for the order that will be here by November 4th."

We reached his office.

"We've tried to call them and increase our order to include seeds for you, but nobody answers the phone."

It was 4:30 in Seattle, and 6:30 at Nycomed Amersham in Illinois, where the seeds were produced.

"We'll call them again the first thing on Monday morning. One person on our staff is helpful in situations like this. He comes in by 7 A.M. Call my nurse, Jean Stewart, on Monday morning at 9:00. We should know then."

"We can't guarantee you seeds," Jean Stewart said, "but we'll do our best. If we can't get your Iodine-125 from our regular supplier, there are other sources we can try. Call me on Monday. Until then I can't make a definite promise."

"We will," Bob said. "9:00 sharp."

"Try to relax until then. You both look exhausted," she said.

We trudged down a long corridor that connected the office building to the hospital and found the lab. More forms needed to be filled out there.

We waited patiently, numb with weariness. I wished Bob had decided to have the EKG and blood work-up done in Atlanta. We could easily have faxed the results to Dr. Ragde's office. Finally Bob's name was called, and we went into an examining room for the EKG.

Bob removed his jacket, tie, shirt, undershirt, shoes, and socks. I had lost count of how many times that day he'd taken off and put on various items of clothing.

An exceptionally pleasant woman did Bob's EKG. She attached electrodes to his hairy chest and his ankles. The electrical current feeds a stylus that records electrical charges passing along different portions of the heart and records them on graph paper.

When the study was completed, she said, "you're not going to like me any more. Those electrodes that went on so easily will hurt coming off. They're attached like glue."

Bob winced as the electrodes came off and took strands of hair with them. Bob dressed again. He looked drained.

Then she led us to the blood lab. I sat outside, because blood work is routine. It was the first time that Bob and I had been separated during a medical procedure since that first ultrasound and biopsy at the urologist's office in Atlanta.

Exhausted and disoriented, we tried to find a taxi. Taxis had been difficult to find at our hotel in the center of downtown. We saw none at Northwest Hospital, at least five miles north of the hub. Bob noticed a man wheeling an ultrasound unit toward a parking lot.

"Where can I find a taxi around here?" Bob asked him.

"I don't know. Where are you going?"

"Downtown to our hotel. The Vintage Park."

"I'm going past downtown. I can pull off at an exit close to your hotel. That is if you two don't mind sharing a single seat in the front of my van. This equipment fills up the back."

"Mind? I'd be thankful beyond telling."

"We're genuinely grateful," I said. "This will be your best good deed of the year."

We'd met yet another friendly Seattleite.

We watched him load the ultrasound unit onto his van by using an electronic fork that slid from the vehicle to the ground. The unit was rolled onto the fork, raised up, then rolled into the van. We all piled into the front.

Driving down the highway, he called his wife and told her about us. We looked like two stranded urchins. But, if he noticed, he didn't mention that. He only told her that he'd be a few minutes late getting home, because he was dropping two people off downtown. He left us a few blocks from the hotel, and we found our weary way there.

I went directly to the reception desk and said, "We need a room from November 1st to November 6th. A junior suite would be nice. If that's not available, put us in 1006 again. It's lovely."

"A suite is available," she said.

"We booked this stay at the club rate. Can we have that rate again?"

"Sure. Matter of fact, you can have the suite for the same price as your present room."

More Seattle kindness. I went to the concierge's desk.

"Greg," I said, "please call Delta airlines for me."

He did, and it took an infernally long time to make the reservations. While on hold, I said to Greg, "No one will be able to reach you. I'm tying up your phone."

"Don't worry."

"You're the kindest concierge I've ever met."

He smiled. By the time the transaction was completed, we had two round-trip tickets at $286 each, with a $50 penalty if we changed the day of the flights in case the radiation seeds couldn't be found.

"Go upstairs and relax," he said. "Come down and drink wine by the fireplace from six to seven."

"Thanks," I said. "We have wine in our room. We'll sip some there."

It was wonderful to kick off our shoes and sink into those deep armchairs with our feet propped up on the ottomans.

"How do you feel, honey?" I asked him.

"Bushed," he answered.

"Not victorious?"

"Not yet."

"Why?"

"Because we don't have the seeds yet."

"Jean Stewart said they'd work on it early Monday morning."

"She also said that she couldn't make a definite promise."

"Be of good cheer." I poured us both a glass of red wine and said, "Here's to Monday when we know they have seeds reserved for you."

"To Monday and to seeds," he said listlessly. "I need a long hot shower."

Bob took a shower and emerged in a terry cloth robe. Looking rosy from the hot water, he sprawled in his chair.

We went to dinner at Tulio at 7:30. We were waiting to be seated when a man came over to us, the same person that Bob had guessed was a southerner at Dr. Ragde's office. He introduced himself and asked if we would join him and his wife for dinner.

I preferred dinner alone, and I guess Bob did, too. But it would have been rude to refuse, so we let him lead us to their table. They were from Nashville. She started to talk about her husband's cancer.

"Look," I said, "We've all been living cancer all day long. Let's not eat it for dinner, too."

"Okay," she agreed.

"You tell us what you like about Nashville, and we'll tell you the same about Atlanta."

They were pleasant dinner companions. By 8:45 we were back in 1006 for a long night's sleep. I didn't even bother to take a shower. We'd pack our few belongings tomorrow. The plane didn't leave until after noon.

The next morning we woke with lively libidos and made extravagant love. We both felt such a sense of relief. We rolled all over that bed. Bob claimed it was the biggest bed he'd ever been in, though in reality it was the same size as our bed at home. We were euphoric, and our euphoria spilled over into our lovemaking.

The flight home was nothing like the gloomy one to Seattle, when I hid from the world by keeping my window shade drawn. I sat by a window with the shade up to admire the view. The clouds were dispersing, and the sun illuminated the mountainous terrain of the Northwest spread out beneath me.

On the yellow legal pad where I usually kept notes about cancer, I wrote:

MOUNT RAINIER

The other mountains are snow-capped too;
clouds hover over them.

But Rainier soars above the clouds
who grovel by her base.

And she reflects with majesty
the glory of the sun.

Not a great poem. Simply visual. Still it felt great to be in a poetry mood again.

BOB

You lose most of a day flying from Seattle to Atlanta. That suited me. I was riveted on Monday morning, nine o'clock in Seattle, noon in Atlanta.

I was also bone tired. We unpacked our few things and flopped into bed. Praise flopped into bed with us. He had seen so little of us these past weeks. We slept exceeding well and woke before nine. We seemed to be on Atlanta time.

We spent Sunday morning in bed with *The New York Times* and *The Atlanta Journal-Constitution.* It felt great to laze in bed and browse through the newspapers. We each drank several mugs of my hazelnut coffee. Praise stretched over newspaper sections and burrowed under them.

We walked our miles outdoors that afternoon. The brilliant sun highlighted the hues of changing leaves on trees. The crisp air energized us. It was indeed a beautiful day.

Monday. Noon in Atlanta, 9 A.M. in Seattle. Saralee listened on the kitchen phone, and I used my desk phone to call Dr. Meier's office and speak with Jean Stewart. The seed order that was sent from Seattle on Friday hadn't been processed. Seeds for me would be included in that order.

Dr. Meier's nurse told us that we needed to arrive in Seattle on Sunday, because we had an appointment at Dr. Ragde's office with Donna at 9:30 A.M. on Monday. The two offices seemed thoroughly coordinated. On Tuesday morning Dr. Ragde and Dr. Meier would do the surgery together.

Saralee ran into my library, and we clung to one another, relieved and jubilant. I would be seeded and safe in two weeks and one day. On the way to total cure.

SARALEE

Since we didn't have enough frequent flyer miles for free tickets, we decided to fly to Seattle on Saturday and take advantage of Delta's reduced weekend rate. We bought tickets. I called the hotel and told them we'd arrive one day earlier than our specified reservation. I asked Greg to make dinner reservations for us, and he did. We'd arrive in Seattle in less than two weeks.

The time in Atlanta sped by. The architectural control committee met each Tuesday at 8 P.M. I could concentrate on these meetings now and enjoy the choices we made.

We took Judith and Mark to Theater Emory for "Lost," Steve Murray's new play. We told them that we had felt as lost as the characters in the play while Bob decided how to treat his cancer. We talked about our gratefulness that this trauma would be behind us soon and about the appropriateness of seeding for Bob.

"What did you think he'd choose?" Mark asked me. "To truncate himself at the waist?"

"Nothing he chose would have surprised me," I said. "And the decision had to be his."

"For sure," Judith said. "If you decided wrong, he'd be a goner."

I thought, we'd both be goners.

"I've heard other men say the hardest part of dealing with prostate cancer is deciding how to treat it," Mark said.

I hoped that Mark was right.

"You bet," Bob said. "Deciding what to do with this wild card was frantic."

Sunday afternoon brought the sadness of attending a memorial service for a friend's husband. During docent training at the museum six years ago, Joan had been my mentor, my big sister, She had been kind, generous, and inspirational. Joan and I remained friends afterwards.

We had partied with Joan and her husband, Ted, a charming and devoted couple. Ted had retired from his medical practice two years before and shared his computer skills generously with Jimmy Carter's Habitat for Humanity and his friends.

Joan and Ted had finally found time to enjoy life together. On Thursday evening they had dinner out with friends. He had a heart attack at 11 P.M. and died immediately. Joan had no time to prepare herself for this ultimate loss.

As she was led down the aisle by her sons, Joan cried. She seemed helpless—innocent, shorn, and bereft. I bit back my tears; Joan was living my worst nightmare.

On Wednesday morning I phoned Dr. Ragde's office to tell them we'd arrive in Seattle on Saturday and to see if they had any last minute instructions for us.

"This is a coincidence," the receptionist said. "We were going to call you on Friday. I'll put Donna on the line."

There was a pause, and then a voice, considerate as Dr. Ragde's but feminine, said, "Hello. I have some medical questions for Dr. Fine. Do you want to answer them or will Dr. Fine call me?"

"After forty years together I can probably answer them," I said.

She asked me routine health questions, which I had no trouble answering. Bob's uneventful health history needed little explanation. The only question that I couldn't answer dealt with tonsillectomy.

"You can assume he had one. Everybody did when we were kids," I said. "Do you want him to call you about that?"

"No. I'll ask about his tonsils when we meet on Monday."

"Okay. Can you think of anything we don't know about and ought to?"

"Yes. Bring a charge card with you on the day of surgery. The pharmacy will accept that as payment and deliver the medications he needs while Dr. Fine is in recovery."

"Thanks. Is there anything else I need to know?"

She thought for a moment then asked, "Has anyone mentioned jockey shorts?"

"No. What about them?"

"Bring some. He'll need them instead of boxer shorts to hold an ice pack, then a pad if he bleeds. He'll like their support after surgery while he's swollen and tender."

"Thanks. We didn't know about that."

I hung up the phone and checked Bob's underwear. He had only four pairs of jockey shorts in his drawer. I called and told him he'd need more.

"Can I buy you some?" I asked.

"Don't bother. I'll pick up some Fruit of the Loom shorts at K-Mart."

"Okay. Donna, who we'll meet on Monday, asked if you'd had your tonsils out. I told her you probably had, but I wasn't sure."

"Yes, when I was ten."

"That's before my time. See you at home, love."

Seattle Again

~

BOB

Saturday's flight to Seattle had many empty seats, so Saralee and I used three seats each. We stretched out during the long flight on banks of seats adjacent to each other. I looked forward to exploring Seattle that weekend and was confident that Tuesday's surgery would go well.

Our plane arrived on time, and we carried our bags through the terminal to a waiting taxi. We arrived at the hotel at 11 A.M., sure that our luggage would need to be stored and surprised that our room was ready.

We moved in and unpacked in a spacious corner room with a view of Mount Rainier. We relaxed briefly from the trip, then we went downstairs and asked Greg where to buy Oregon and Washington wines.

"Go to De Laurenti's in the Pike Place market," he said. "Talk to Joe. He's knows wine and will help you choose."

Saralee was delighted that we were heading for Pike Place. She had read about flower stands there and planned to buy a bouquet.

The crisp weather made our walk to the market pleasant. Saralee bought dahlias from the first stand we passed. We found De Laurenti's Specialty Foods nearby. A man cutting Italian cheeses directed us to the wine department upstairs, where we asked for Joe.

"You're speaking to him," Joe said.

"We want some Oregon and Washington red wines," I said.

We followed him down narrow aisles and helped him select our wines. Each of us carried a bag of wine to the hotel along with the dahlias.

Greg found a vase for the flowers, and Saralee arranged them on a table in our sitting area. We could see them from our bed or anywhere else we sat. We relaxed in our attractive home-away-from-home. It was a beautiful day.

As we walked down steep hills to a restaurant, we held hands, not so much for emotional support, but out of simple affection. I had never felt closer to her. She'd been a brick while I made my decision. A simple procedure would soon begin my cure. Until then we owed ourselves the pleasures of Seattle.

We ate a simple lunch. We had planned to walk along the waterfront after lunch but found ourselves tired. Instead we napped all afternoon.

We stopped in the lobby to taste Columbia wines before dinner. Saralee liked the white. She said the chardonnay was full of apple aroma.

Dinner delighted Saralee. She ordered an appetizer of thirteen different raw oysters and said that would be plenty for her. I ate salmon, the house specialty. We chose two different beers and shared each. We sat close and touched frequently. Though I ate no oysters, they served as our aphrodisiac.

SARALEE

We woke on Sunday morning to full sun. The morning usually began hazily in Seattle, and the sun broke through later. Mount Rainier stood regally in the distance. We ate breakfast in bed. Bob spooned his way through a soup bowl of steaming oatmeal topped with brown sugar and raisins. The black decaf coffee was plenty for me.

We planned to walk all day. First we stopped at SAM to see Leonardo daVinci Rediscovered. The ticket seller remembered us from the last trip. The jammed exhibition rooms made us use a strategy to avoid traffic. Instead of moving with the crowd around the room, we moved in the opposite direction. That way we didn't wait in line to see the next work.

We viewed at our own pace, sometimes lingering at works that delighted us, sometimes bypassing others entirely. We found the 20th-century renditions of daVinci's famous paintings exciting because of the innovative ways that the originals had been reinterpreted. Then we explored the museum's 20th century collection. These uncrowded galleries allowed more elbow room for leisurely viewing.

We'd brought a hamper with wine and checked it at the coat room. Later we'd sit in a park and enjoy a glassful. When we claimed our wine, the attendant told us that the bottle had tipped and most of the wine was gone. We explained the bottle hadn't been full to begin with. With typical Seattle kindness, he insisted on refunding the full bottle price.

We sauntered along First Avenue toward the international district.

BOB

As soon as we turned the bend on First Avenue, the aromas of garlic and spices surrounded us. I enjoy ethnicity, so does Saralee. We strolled through shops but bought nothing, until Saralee found an Asian grocery store with sweet red peppers; she bought two beauties.

When we reached Occidental Park, we sat on a bench and sipped the skimpy remainder of wine. The trees, luminous with sun, delighted us. We saw Japanese wall sculptures, radiant at noon.

A street person with a hand-rolled cigarette asked us for a light. His clothes smelled of marihuana. We told him that we had no matches. He sat with us anyhow and talked about his father, a doctor who had died of lung cancer. Intelligent and articulate, he'd dropped out of college. Now he claimed that he was starved for the company of intellectuals.

We roamed the neighborhood until we found Sea Garden, where we'd eat lunch. All of the customers were Asian at this authentic restaurant, except for us. I ordered more Chinese food than we could eat. We had left no room for dessert, but they brought us the traditional cookies.

Saralee opened a cookie and read me her fortune, "Now, it is best to take things one step at a time."

"It's a beautiful day," I replied.

After lunch we explored the Danny Woo International District Community Garden nearby. We climbed steps on which we read,

> May each step
> you take
> and each seed
> you sow
> bring you closer
> to prosperity
> and happiness.

We meandered along the Alaskan Way at the waterfront. To the north were snow-capped mountains. We strolled south and stopped to watch, as ferries disgorged vehicles and passengers, then inhaled people and cars.

We climbed steep flights of stairs, at various angles to one another. At the top, we were surprised to find ourselves at the Pike Street market. Saralee saw a stand with local chantarelles. In addition to being addicted to oysters, she's a mushroom freak.

"Wow," she said. "I want to buy some before we leave Seattle and take them back home with us. We can't afford what they cost in Atlanta."

We left the market and strolled along Pike Place. A bakery displayed chocolate dusted meringues. The smells of sugar, chocolate, and fruit fillings made me salivate. Limitless varieties of puff pastry beguiled me. I selected rich pastries for later that evening plus a stuffed croissant and a raisin roll for my breakfast. Monday's breakfast would be my last meal until after surgery. I'd subsist on a liquid diet from then on.

We became so comfortable in our room that we canceled our dinner reservation. We had meringues and eclairs for snacks. What we wanted was white wine. We called Greg.

"May we come downstairs and get two glasses of the Columbia white you'll be pouring later?" I asked. "We're so lazy that we're staying home tonight."

"You don't need to come downstairs for the wine," he said. "I'll bring you some."

He knocked at our door few minutes later with a whole bottle of wine in an ice bucket.

"Wow," I said. "You didn't need to bring that much."

"I wanted to," he replied. "Enjoy it."

SARALEE

Monday's weather, penetratingly cold, alternated between mist and rain. We took a taxi to Dr. Ragde's office for our appointment with Donna. She handed us a paper with instructions for follow-up care after surgery. It could be done by a local urologist, except that Dr. Ragde would examine Bob one year after surgery and do a biopsy at 18 months. Bob asked if his Atlanta urologist could do the one year exam. Donna suggested that we let Dr. Ragde decide. She told us to plan on coming back in 18 months; Dr. Ragde didn't want anyone else tinkering around with his surgery. He'd do his own biopsy. We understood and agreed.

Donna was everyone's ideal mother. She asked if we knew where to go for surgery tomorrow. We knew. She asked if Bob remembered about his liquid diet before surgery. He remembered. She told us his surgery had been changed to 11 A.M., so Bob could drink coffee until 8. The surgery would last about 45 minutes. He'd stay until he was "street fit" and could walk. We'd leave, somewhere between 1 and 2 P.M. Donna's reassuring demeanor made us feel relaxed the day before surgery.

Dr. Ragde came out of his office and shook hands with us.

"I have some questions to ask you," he said to Bob. "Follow me."

He led us to a lecture hall. The equipment for seed implantation was shown on a table in the hallway outside. I saw the grey metal template that was used to place the implants evenly, marked A, B, C, D, E, F, G horizontally and numbered vertically. The holes between the marks were one centimeter apart. Dark pellets, the length of a grain of rice, only more slender, sat beside the template.

The long needles frightened me. I hoped that Bob hadn't noticed them. If he had, he didn't talk about the needles, and I mentioned nothing about them.

We listened, as Dr. Ragde explained the seeding process to a group of physicians. They would spend today learning about implant surgery and watch, on closed circuit television, as Dr. Ragde did the implants tomorrow.

Afterwards we followed Dr. Ragde back to his office. His lion's mane of hair was slicked back today. He wore a smart pink shirt, a maroon tie with diagonal stripes, dark trousers, a starched lab coat, and his reliable rubber-bottomed shoes. He sat at his desk; we, on the sofa opposite. He asked questions and wrote Bob's answers on a legal pad.

"Has anyone in your immediate family ever had prostate cancer?" he asked.

"No," Bob answered.

"Good. Has anyone in your immediate family had any other form of cancer?"

"No."

"Have you ever had surgery on your prostate gland?"

"No."

"Good. How many times a night do you wake to urinate?"

"Once. But my stream is weaker."

"It happens to all of us as we get older," he said.

"When was your last PSA?"

"August 8th, this year."

"What was the level?"

"3.7"

"Have you had an MRI or CT to help diagnose your cancer?"

"An MRI."

"Have you had a bone scan?"

"No, an acid phosphatase that came back normal."

"Has anyone been able to feel a nodule?"

"No."

"Good. Okay, then we're set for tomorrow."

He rose, came around the desk, and we shook hands again.

We had gathered a list of radio cabs from the hotel. I called one from the office desk. We walked to the door, then waited inside, away from the cold and damp, until the taxi came.

"Why did he ask you all those questions?" I asked Bob. "He knows those things."

"He's making a formal record for future research of what was there at the beginning," Bob told me.

BOB

We shopped for my liquid groceries with my umbrella over us. We found a take-out shop with orange juice, Snaffle, and bottled sparkling water a few blocks from the hotel. I'd want hot broth in this weather. We should have left the heavy liquid containers at the store, while we searched for bouillon cubes and something for Saralee to eat. We could have picked them up on the way back to the hotel.

Instead we carried them with us. Saralee insisted she'd carry the bag if I held the umbrella. When her arms ached later, she rotated the load with me.

We found salt-free bouillon cubes and a lemon to slice into hot water at De Laurenti's. Saralee chose two pieces of cheese. She'd eat them with the sweet red peppers we'd bought yesterday. She didn't buy bread, because she knew that bread would be too tempting for me.

Saralee chose a bunch of dried flowers to replace the wilted dahlias. She was determined that our room remain cheerful during the next few days. We returned to the shelter of our hotel and relaxed until the weather cleared. We shared sunset, as the radio played Handel's Water Music.

On Tuesday at 8 A.M. I stopped drinking coffee and gave myself an enema. It produced fewer cramps than I had experienced with former enemas, probably because of my 24 hour liquid diet.

I felt anxious in the taxi. I hoped my doctors were feeling well today. I hoped that they would aim well. When we left the expressway and came to Meridian Avenue, we turned left toward outpatient surgery, rather than right toward the hospital.

We entered a waiting room with a long curved desk and clerks. Saralee and I sat together, while I filled out consent forms. I would permit hospitalization, diagnostic tests, and therapy done by my physicians or their assistants. I consented to blood transfusions if necessary. I sure hoped that I wouldn't need any.

I gave permission for the hospital to release all medical informa-tion needed to facilitate payment for my care. I agreed to the release of any information needed for post-discharge care. I certified that I was eligible for Medicare and requested that payments be made.

I authorized Dr. Ragde and his associates or assistants to treat my prostate carcinoma. I asserted the procedure planned was a prostate seed implant with ultrasound.

I acknowledged that during the course of surgery or after surgery unforseen circumstances might occur and other procedures might be necessary. I hoped that wouldn't happen to me either. I authorized Dr. Ragde and his team to do anything necessary if it happened.

I consented to anesthesia and its possible complications, includ-ing damage to major organs, cardiac arrest, paralysis, or brain death. This didn't rattle me. Patients sign their consent for that whenever I inject contrast material for CT scans.

I gave permission to take and reproduce photographs, moving pictures, and closed circuit television pictures during my surgery. I consented to their use afterwards for educational purposes.

I acknowledged that I knew I was facing significant risks and that no guarantee had been given me as to result or cure.

When I had finished signing myself away, a clerk clipped a patient identification bracelet on my arm. A nurse led me to a changing room, a tiny cubicle with one shelf to sit on while I removed my clothes. I had already given Saralee my wallet and wrist-watch.

The nurse handed me a hospital gown, paper slippers, and a plastic bag for my clothing, labeled with my name and Dr. Ragde's. She pointed out where to go when I'd finished changing. I closed the cubicle curtain, put on the patient's gown and slippers, and left my bag of personal belongings in the room. I assumed that they would be stored until I could use them again.

I shuffled down the hall in paper slippers, and opened the door to a huge room, subdivided with curtains that could be pulled shut. I saw Saralee and went to her. Officially a patient now, I sat in a reclining chair beside her.

"Are you okay?" she asked.

"Sure," I lied, the nervous center of attention lounging in his chair.

My bag of personal belongings was delivered, and Saralee took it.

"A catheter is going to be put into your vein," a nurse explained A tech followed.

"This will be easy for you," I said. "I have big veins."

The tech injected enough Novocain to raise a pimple under my skin. The Novocain masked all pain as she inserted the catheter into a vein on top of my left hand. She taped the catheter in place.

The anesthesiologist came into my cubicle and introduced himself.

"I'll do a spinal on you for surgery," he said. "Do you have any allergies?"

"I have a questionable allergy to penicillin," I said. "Nothing else."

"Okay."

"I'm anxious about this," I volunteered. "Could you give me some sedation?"

"Sure, we frequently do that. Some people want to observe as much as possible. Others don't."

"I don't want to be totally unconscious."

"No, I wouldn't do that to you."

He left, and Saralee squeezed my right hand, the one without the catheter.

"I asked for sedation, because I can't help out during surgery," I said.

"That's for sure," she told me. "Just lie still and let it happen."

"I'll be better off relaxed."

A nurse told me that they were finishing up the case before me in the operating room and would be ready for me in ten or fifteen minutes.

Saralee told the nurse that she wanted to watch my surgery. The nurse informed Saralee that this was against administration policy. Only one other woman had ever wanted to go into the operating room with her husband.

Saralee explained that she didn't want to be in the operating room. She wanted to watch through the closed-circuit television set-up with the doctors learning the procedure. She told the nurse that she was writing a book about prostate cancer. Being able to describe my surgery was essential. The nurse said that Saralee needed written approval by the hospital's attorney in administration. There wasn't time for that.

Dr. Meier came to my chair and said, "Do you remember me?"

"Of course I remember you, Dr. Meier," I answered. "Scrubs and a surgical cap aren't enough to disguise you."

Dr. Ragde came to us.

"Please let me watch Bob's surgery on closed-circuit television," Saralee pleaded. "I have to know what the surgery looks like."

"What makes you want that?" Dr. Ragde asked.

"We're writing about our experience at Northwest Hospital and about you and Dr. Meier. Bob will be sedated and unaware of what's happening. Please let me watch, so I can record his surgery."

Sympathetic, Dr. Ragde readily agreed. There was no time for administrative forms. A nurse handed him a blank sheet of paper and a pen, and Dr. Ragde wrote an informal consent.

"You go there," Dr. Ragde told Saralee and pointed to a door. "You can have a cup of coffee while you watch."

"Thanks," she said and smiled gratefully. "I don't need coffee. I promise you a beautiful book."

SARALEE

A nurse wheeled Bob away, and I went toward the door that Dr. Ragde had indicated. Dianna Lynn Davis, the nurse manager, accompanied me and sat beside me, close to the television. A table full of sandwiches separated us from the doctors who also observed the TV. Suzi Hedrick Beerman, the media and public-relations coordinator for Northwest Hospital, joined us. She gave me a thick packet of information to read later and sat down on my other side.

I was both scared and fascinated. Later I told Bob that I felt like oozy peanut butter and jelly, supported by Dianna and Suzi, two stable slabs of bread.

The television screen was divided into sections. The top right showed an enlarged picture of a prostate gland, implanted with dark pellets.

"That's the last patient's gland," Dianna Davis explained. "When they're done, your husband's prostate will be shown there."

"Is it okay if I put my recorder near the TV?" I asked.

"Sure," she said.

I watched as Bob's feet were placed in stirrups. A tube was inserted into his rectum, and clear liquid rushed out.

"What's that?" I asked.

"The residue of fluid in his lower colon," the nurse said. "The drainage tube is orange."

"Spare me the colorful details," I said. "When Bob was an intern, he took me into the emergency room with him. Only once. I passed out when I saw the bright red blood. I was more of a problem than the patient."

"Really?" Suzi asked.

"Definitely. I'm relieved that this TV shows only black and white. Blood makes me woozy. There's no telling how Bob's blood will affect me. Will he bleed much?"

"Some, but probably not a lot," Dianna said.

"Don't worry," Suzi said and patted my hand. "We're staying here to see you through this. You and your husband are going to get through surgery A-okay."

"He's had a spinal," Dianna said. "The sedation he asked for is taking effect. He can't feel a thing."

"What are they putting on him now?" I asked.

"Betadine. It's an antiseptic. He's already been prepped," Dianna said.

Bob was liberally doused with Betadine. His scrotum and penis were encased in plastic.

"I wish they were wrapping his privates in lead—just to be sure nothing happens to them," I said.

"He's doing fine," Suzi said. "He has the best urologic surgeon for this procedure in the world."

Bob's penis and scrotal sac were raised and taped to his abdomen with his perineum clearly visible for surgery. All I could see on the TV was the lower half of Bob, mainly his perineum.

I watched as the gigantic dildo of an ultrasound probe went into Bob's rectum. I thought, let this be the last time any probe is jammed into him.

I couldn't see Bob's face to know whether he could feel anything.

"Are you sure he doesn't hurt?" I asked Dianna.

"Positive," she said. "Relax."

I believed Dianna. I had delivered both our daughters under spinal anesthesia and had never felt any pain.

I could hear doctors' voices behind me in the closed-circuit TV room. I turned and looked at them briefly and noticed that fewer were here than had attended the lecture the day before.

"Where are all the doctors I saw yesterday?" I asked.

"Some of them are in the operating room to observe the surgery first hand," the nurse said.

"Will Dr. Ragde be able to concentrate on Bob?"

"Of course," Dianna said and squeezed my hand. "He does this all the time. He knows perfectly well how to operate and lecture at the same time."

"What's that beeping sound?" I asked.

"They're monitoring your husband's pulse," Dianna said. "It's done by sound. That way, his doctors don't have to look up to know how he's doing. They can concentrate on the surgery."

"That lets them pay more attention to your husband," Suzi said.

"Do you hear how regular the beeps are?" Dianna asked.

"Yes," I said.

"That means his pulse is steady. He's doing fine."

I could hear more than I could see. The camera was aimed at Bob's perineum. I could see nothing else in the operating room. A metal grid was placed over Bob's perineum.

"You can watch the whole thing here," Dr. Ragde said to Bob. "Be sure we do the right thing. Okay?"

Later Bob told me that there was a mirror, and he could watch the surgery.

I'd hear a nurse say a word and a number.

"What do the words and numbers mean?" I asked Dianna.

"The words—Baker, Charley, Delta, Echo, Frank, and so forth—refer to the letters A, B, C, D, E, F, G on the horizontal sides of the template. The numbers refer to numbers on the vertical side of the template."

Dr. Ragde repeated the word and number to verify that he had heard accurately. Then he inserted a needle. The back of Dr. Ragde's head, covered with a surgical cap, was all I could see when the needle went in. That suited me fine. I'd never know how deep the needles went into Bob.

"I saw the needles yesterday," I said. "They're long and scary."

"Dr. Ragde knows just how to place them," Suzi said. "He's done this procedure thousands of times before."

After a number of needles had been placed and removed, I saw blood seeping from the template.

"How much blood is he losing?" I asked. "Will he need a transfusion?"

"He has hardly lost any blood at all," Dianna said. "The blood is barely oozing. It would be rare to need a transfusion with this minor procedure."

"Blood isn't as frightening shown in black and white instead of technicolor red," I said. "I'm nowhere near fainting."

"Good," they said simultaneously.

I began to think of Bob as a human pincushion with long, sharp pins penetrating deep into his body. I kept wishing that the surgery would end. That it would be over quickly. That Bob would be past danger.

Because Dr. Ragde was teaching, he talked as he did Bob's surgery. He'd repeat a description of what was happening with each needle he inserted.

"We do it right there, and then we pull it back. We can't see it on ultrasound. Move forward so we can see it again, the tip of the needle, and back again and back forward. And now we can barely see it. Go back a millimeter, push the stylet forward. We push out the bone wax. And there is the first seed sitting exactly where we wanted it. And we drop the seeds in spaces in a row."

Dr. Ragde's voice sounded wonderful—calm, instructive, and gentle. Listening to him, I became less frightened about Bob and more interested in the surgery itself.

"Tell me what Dr. Ragde is doing," I said to Dianna.

The nurse explained that a blunt-tipped stylet sat inside the hollow needle. Wax sat between the stylet and the seeds. When Dr. Ragde pushed the stylet in, wax was pushed forward. The wax pushed the seeds into the gland in a row.

"Is this process repeated over and over, until all of Bob's prostate is seeded?" I asked.

"Exactly," Dianna said. "The surgery continues until all of his gland is evenly seeded."

I heard a nurse say that an adjustment was needed.

"What's wrong?" I asked.

"Sometimes the prostate swells during the surgery," Dianna said. "They need a new starting place, a new top of the prostate."

I heard Dr. Meier's voice, but couldn't make out the words.

"What did Dr. Meier say?" I asked.

"Dr. Meier is talking about the changing width of Bob's gland. The nurse alerted him to check that and make any needed alteration. The surgery is a team effort."

"We're really getting a good job here," Dr. Ragde said.

"Well, I traveled this far," Bob said.

"He sounds quite alert," I said.

"Yes," Suzi agreed. "Perky."

"Are they close to finishing?" I asked.

"Yes," Dianna said.

She explained that there were lots of implanted seeds now and various densities in the gland itself. The numerous seeds could confuse the ultrasound image. The only way to identify the current needle was to watch what moves on ultrasound. We couldn't see that from where we were.

"I expected to cry," I said to them. "All I can feel is gratitude that this is being done for us."

"You'll cry later—from relief," Dianna said. "Look, they're almost done."

"Well, we're going to take a walk now and see what this looks like," Dr. Ragde said. "Fluoro, please."

Fluoro meant fluoroscopy, a type of X-ray image that moves, rather than a stationary picture.

"A beautiful implant," Dr. Ragde said.

I laughed and continued laughing. I was filled with a rush of joy and relief that surgery had been completed. On the upper left of the television screen, Bob's prostate appeared, his grey gland studded with darker pellets.

"Isn't he gorgeous?" I said. "And that's how he'll look forever and ever."

"Let's take a look again," Dr. Ragde said.

"It looks more concentrated on the left than the right," Bob said.

I was still chuckling.

"No, it's fine," Dr. Ragde said.

"You can't tell by looking at this," Dr. Meier said. "It's just sort of an idea."

"Right," Bob said. "It's only two-dimensional."

"But you get a CT scan tomorrow," Dr. Ragde said.

A CT scan is three-dimensional.

"How far into the capsule did you go?" Bob asked.

"We go right into the capsule," Dr. Ragde said. "The effective radiation is 5 millimeters beyond the capsule."

"Thank you very much," Bob said.

Still laughing, I said, "He's very alert now."

"Yes, his sedation has worn off," Dianna said, "but the spinal is still effective. He's feeling no pain."

I watched as his scrotum and penis were unwrapped. His penis was weeping. Something thicker than water, something viscous. I wondered if it were semen.

"Do you want to try it without a catheter?" Dr. Ragde asked Bob.

"I'd love to," Bob said.

"Okay," Dr. Ragde said.

"I'm so happy it's over," I said and moved the recorder back to Dianna, Suzi, and me.

"He's fine," Dianna said. "Now the nurses will clean him up and transfer him to the recovery room. As soon as they get the first set of vital signs and what not, you and I can go in there, and you can see him."

"I'd like that a lot," I said.

I felt as if we'd been connected vicariously by TV forever. I wanted to see him and know he felt okay. I wanted to be near him, so I could touch him again.

"What nobody sees is that we'll run the Geiger counter over the table, over everything," Dianna said. "We have to account for every seed that was brought into the room, all 99 of them."

"They are very thorough with follow-up when radioactive seeds are involved," Suzi said.

"The same thing applies once you're in the recovery room," Dianna continued. "The room is scanned. The bedding is scanned."

"That is precise," I said.

"When you go to get your discharge instructions, you'll get a little strainer for the urine."

"Thank you," I said and hoped that all the seeds would stay exactly where Dr. Ragde had placed them.

"You're the person who's helping me most," Suzi said to me.

She was referring to our book. If it were published, the book would boost the hospital where she does public relations.

"She helps me all the time," the nurse said. "I know that she's great."

Though the picture of the operating room was disconnected, the sound was still on. I heard the same sort of jubilation that we felt coming from there, that surge of relief when surgery is complete.

"Do you have any questions?" Suzi asked.

"Really not," I said. "Bob taught me so much. I just needed to see the actual process."

"Did you know what to expect?"

"I had a pretty good idea, because we were here yesterday," I said. "We sat in while Dr. Ragde talked with the doctors studying here, and we saw the template. We saw the seeds."

"Okay, so you really knew what to expect," Suzi said. "That's great. A good education. Even some medical people don't care about that."

"It will be a narrative told by a couple in love," I said. "It will not be merely technical."

"If it's for patients, it usually doesn't have to have the level of detail . . . ." Dianna said.

"I understand. Northwest Hospital's booklet, "Seeds of Hope, Seeds of Health," helped me. It put the doctors' technical terms into lay language."

"Right. That's why we wrote it," Suzi said.

"Our forty-year-old marriage is an important part of the book. We're twin voices coaxing each other over thin ice."

"Who's your publisher?"

"We'll have to see who wants this kind of book."

"I would say the need for it is pretty high," Suzi said. "You should get some takers there. I'm going to leave you now."

"Okay."

"If you need anything at all, I'll be back in my office."

" 'Bye," Dianna said and turned to me. "As soon as they get him set up in the next room, I'll escort you there. I'm writing, too. When my article gets published, I'll send you a copy."

"That would be fabulous," I said. "But our book is not all that technical."

"When I lecture, I also stress what this couple has gone through to get to this point. Their stress and struggles."

"Yes."

"When you have almost 200,000 men in the U.S. diagnosed in 1997, that's a lot of people."

"How many?"

"200,000."

"Wow. I had no idea prostate cancer was that widespread."

"And 40,000 prostate-cancer deaths. I'm going to the recovery room to see if he's ready."

When she returned, Dianna motioned me to follow her. She led me to Bob, who lay in his recliner covered with a blanket. On a stand above him, an intravenous traveled through a tube to the catheter in his hand.

I was elated to see him, but I was afraid to touch him. I was afraid to jar the IV or hurt some part of him hidden beneath the blanket.

"Do you need another blanket?" a nurse asked him.

"No, I'm doing fine," he answered.

He sounded so matter-of-fact, his usual laid-back self. Dianna introduced me to his nurse, Shannon.

"This is Mrs. Fine," she said.

"Hi," I said.

"When all this is said and done, she's going to write a book."

"Over a hundred pages are written already."

"Oh really," Shannon said.

"Yes."

"She was able to view this, and she's been doing some recording," Dianna said.

"I still am," I said. "Is that okay?"

"Sure," Shannon said.

Both nurses left. We were alone. I wanted to hug him but was still afraid that I'd hurt him. Hugs would have to wait.

"Did you watch me on TV?" Bob asked me.

"Yes, you're a mini-series. I could see you the whole time. Well, just your perineum. Not even that when the needles went in. Just Dr. Ragde's head. He's the star."

"It went beautifully, I think. Beautiful spinal. Umm. I got a little sedation, not too much."

"I know. I heard you talking."

"I didn't say much."

I laughed and said, "Honey, no one was asking you to say anything at all."

"Yes, really. Now this is all finished. All this preparation and research and talking and everything. And now that's done. My PSA is dropping already."

I laughed, glad to find him lighthearted, the guy I knew before this turmoil began.

"You can feel it, huh?" I asked.

"Hey, it's dropping down."

"Your PSA was within normal range to begin with," I said, laughing.

Shannon came in and asked, "Can I get you some juice?"

"Anything," he said.

"Apple, orange, cranberry."

"Orange would be great. Thank you."

"Sure. I'll be right back."

"It's really strange," he said quietly. "Being the center of all this attention."

I laughed and said, "Soon, we're going to waltz out of here and waltz back into our own lives."

"It went beautifully. I don't think we have to worry."

Shannon returned with a can of juice and a straw that bends stuck in it.

"Thank you," Bob said. "I discovered years ago that when we give patients barium, I always put the straw in upside down."

"Why?" Shannon asked.

"Because if you do, see here?"

"Uh huh."

"It can lead down. But if you put it in the other way, the end is always pointing upward. Here, I'll show you what I mean."

He reversed the ends of the straw.

The nurse laughed and said, "Well, I'll remember that little trick."

"We don't spill barium that way."

"Do you want a sandwich?"

"Sure, please."

She left to get it.

"I'm a little silly, I know."

"Better silly than sad."

"Before you got here, I tried standing. Two nurses helped me. I was woozy. Not my head. My legs. "

"You need to give the spinal time to wear off."

He was his usual impatient self. In a big hurry to get something done.

"Oh Saralee, my legs are so funny. They are so light."

"Because of the anesthesia."

"I know, but it's strange. They're light as can be. It's like I'm floating, like I'm on the moon."

"Here comes a sandwich for you," I said, and Shannon handed him a half sandwich wrapped in transparent plastic.

"Great, thanks," Bob said.

"You're welcome. Best of luck."

"Thanks," we both said.

"Hey," another nurse said. "We're going to let that spinal wear off a little, and then we'll get you up in this chair. Okay?"

"Sure."

"Would you like some water as well as juice?" she asked.

"No. But I'll take another juice in a little while."

"Okay. We have lots of juice. Can I get you some juice?" she asked me.

"Thank you, but no. I might have some wine though if that's permissible."

"Umm, I don't know. I'm sure it would be okay."

"I'd like a glass of wine."

"To celebrate."

She and I both laughed. She left us alone together to celebrate.

"That brought her up," Bob said.

"Unquestionably," I said, as I opened a plastic tote and poured wine into a plastic glass. "Watching this happen, sitting there and watching your surgery, I didn't panic. I didn't cry. All I could feel was gratitude."

Bob ate his sandwich and drank juice. I sipped wine. Classical music was playing in the background, along with sounds of activity— nurses, doctors, presurgical and postsurgical patients.

"Okay," the nurse said. "Here's another orange juice for you."

"Can you get me another sandwich?" Bob asked.

"I don't know."

"There's a table full of sandwiches in the room with the closed-circuit television," I said.

"I'll see," she said and left.

She returned with a whole sandwich, fat with goodies, more juice, and a table to put them on.

"Thanks," we both said.

He reached for the recorder.

"Can I put this on the table?" he asked.

"Certainly."

"Comments," he said, pontificating. "Post-operative comments."

He wanted to take control again. That was fine with me.

"They really run an efficient set-up here. Of course, they've done a few. The anesthesiologist went to school in Atlanta. At Emory."

"Oh really."

"There were quite a few people in the room."

"Yes."

"They think they might have gotten one seed into the base of a seminal vesicle."

"What does a seminal vesicle mean?" I asked, having forgotten some of what he taught me in the flurry of surgery.

"A vesicle holds something. Seminal, semen. It stores semen. Can you remember it that way?"

He held up his juice can and said, "This is a vesicle for orange juice."

"Will your vesicle still store semen?"

"Oh, sure. They got one seed maybe right at it. Anyway, there are two of them. Two seminal vesicles."

"Oh."

"And they're not functional at my age. I don't need semen stored. It has nothing to do with having an orgasm."

He sipped juice.

"I'm still a little dizzy. I think it's from that medication. Sedation."

"I understand."

"I saw one man, as I was being wheeled in here. He must have been number two. I was number three on the schedule. He might have been in street clothes. It's hard to remember."

"Um hmm."

"Anyway, he was sitting up in the chair. That's my next step."

"Yes," I said and thought, there's no hurry.

"They did not put a catheter in me, in my bladder. We're going to try and do it without a catheter."

"I'm happy about that. They put something like a catheter in your rectum before the surgery started."

"That was the ultrasound."

"Before they put the ultrasound in. Bobby, I was sitting there, watching."

"I didn't see any catheter go in the rectum."

"You may have been out of it. Spinal. Sedation."

"Oh, yes. I didn't feel it. I didn't see it either."

"It was there. Dianna, the nurse who was with me, said it was orange."

"I didn't feel them use any antiseptic either. But I'm sure they used it."

"Dianna said they used Betadine. She and Suzi, from public relations, stayed with me the whole time. They were very supportive. Informative, too."

"Yes. Betadine is brownish."

"I couldn't see the color. The TV was black and white."

I didn't say anything about how I felt when I saw him bleeding.

Bob was lifting both his legs and holding them straight out in front of him.

"Is that making you wake up a little better?" a passing nurse asked.

"Well, I don't know. I'm just exercise-conscious."

Bob hoped his leg raises would speed his recovery from the spinal.

"It's coming back. The feeling in my legs."

"It's a beautiful Tuesday."

"Oh, it really is."

"The most beautiful day ever."

"The best."

"Do you hurt?"

"No. Not at all. Not at all. And you're okay?"

I nodded.

"It was a good job. That's why we traveled so far."

"Dr. Fine," Dr. Meier said.

He was between cases.

"Hey, hi," Bob said.

"Looks like it went well," Dr. Meier said. "Nice to see you again," he said to me.

"Hello," I chirped, happy as any bird had ever been.

"It went great," the doctor said. "It was perfect."

Dr. Meier's enthusiasm mirrored our post-surgical high, a heightened vitality that we all shared.

"Did it look like a pretty even distribution?" Bob asked.

"I heard what you mentioned. You never see an absolutely symmetrical distribution. You're looking down with fluoroscopy. It's not a three-dimensional representation. That's why we do the CT."

"Yes, okay."

"But that looks good."

"If the dose goes about half a centimeter, are some of the seeds in the capsule itself?" Bob asked.

"Yes. Some of them are just a few millimeters outside of the prostate."

"I see."

"A few to maybe half a centimeter outside of it."

"Okay."

"Do you know me?" Dr. Ragde asked, as he entered our cubicle.

This scene came straight out of "The Wizard of Oz," as Dorothy meets her lion after each had been transformed by the wizard. But my lion wore surgical scrubs, and a green cap covered his mane. He had done the wizardry himself.

I hugged him and said, "I'll be grateful to you every day—for the rest of my life."

He handed me a packet of information.

"Take it home with you to share with people," Dr. Ragde said.

"Thank you. I'll share this information by using it to write the book," I said.

"It is so organized around here," Bob said. "Everyone is so nice."

"I couldn't see your face during the surgery," I said to Dr. Ragde. "All I saw was the back of your head. But I heard your voice."

"Yuh."

His wonderful voice—decisive, instructive, kind, humble. Dr.

Ragde left, and Dr. Meier continued to brief us.

"There are so many people who come to watch this procedure," he said."

"Yes," Bob said.

"And then there were a lot of people watching on TV, too," I said.

"Right. Exactly," Dr. Meier said and turned to Bob. "Okay, the seeds are in or just outside the prostate."

"Okay. If there's a little invasion outside of the prostate, that would be picked up, too?"

"That is the idea. Yes."

"Okay."

"My job is to draw a prostate treatment volume. Even if the prostate is here . . . "

Dr. Meier described a size by closing one hand.

" . . . we draw the volume a little bigger. You see what I'm saying?"

"Yes."

"So then the dosimetrist decides on the seed distribution, and that's how you treat that. So the prostate treatment is a little larger than the actual prostate itself."

"Good. That makes me feel safe."

"It's the little nuances that happen behind the scenes that you don't know about. We prescribed 16,000 rads."

"Wow. That much makes me feel even safer."

"Let's see. What else? We're going to give you a bunch of literature. It's going to tell you about the medicines."

"I already have that. I started to read it."

"If you don't mind, I just want to ask you a couple of questions."

"Sure."

"We'll give you a few medications. One of them is Bactrim. Do you have any allergies?"

"Just questionably to penicillin."

"Okay. We do that as a preventive. You'll take Bactrim for a week. Do you take any high-blood-pressure medicine?

"No. I had, and I think it made me impotent. I went off of it, and my pressure came to pretty much normal."

"Good."

"When your nurse took my pressure the first time I was here, it was up. But that was one of the most anxious days I've ever had in my whole life."

"Well, the reason I ask you that is that we routinely give patients who have had this procedure either Hytrin or Cardura. It relaxes the smooth muscle in the prostate and allows the urine flow to be better."

"Okay."

"Some people will get a little bit of light-headedness when they take it. So, we recommend that they take it before bedtime."

"Okay.

"It's generally an orthostatic problem."

Orthostatic means standing straight up. The lowered blood pressure would be less apparent if one were lying down.

"You know, when you get up quickly, you might get a little dizzy. But we start with half a pill, and then you go up to one pill a day of Cardura. Take that for a month."

"Oh, for a whole month," Bob said.

"Yes."

"Will it make me impotent?"

"Well, it might affect your sexual function. But then, we'll take you off it."

Neither of us spoke. Impotence was not an issue we wanted to confront.

"Sorry. Cardura helps your bladder. It's possible it could have some other sort of a side effect, too. Some of those blood-pressure medications will."

"Right."

"And it's variable on different people. But the reason we do this is that one out of ten patients will get some constriction of the urinary flow and need to have a catheter. This will diminish the likelihood that you'll need to have a catheter placed."

"Okay."

"What's going to happen is that you're going to have a little bit of soreness in the area where the needles were placed. And you might get a bruise there. It might migrate down to the scrotum or penis. But that will go away. In a few days you'll be feeling pretty much back to normal."

"Good."

"But then, after three, four, five days, you'll start getting symptoms from the seeds themselves, from the radiation."

"Yes."

"And you'll start having urinary frequency. You'll probably get some burning when you urinate. You'll have some urgency. And you will probably have a diminished stream."

"Oh."

"For the diminished stream we just talked about, the Cardura will be a prophylactic. We'll put you on that."

A prophylactic is something that prevents a problem before it begins.

"The other thing we recommend you take is Aleve. You can buy it over the counter.

"Okay."

"The bottle says not to take one more than one, two or three times a day, because it's an over-the-counter medicine. But you can actually take two, twice a day."

"Okay."

"So that's what you should take. Two Aleve twice a day. With something to eat. If you've ever had a problem with gastritis, you may want to take it with a peptic."

A peptic helps digestion.

"Pepcid AC. You can buy them over the counter. But if you don't have any problem with your stomach, just take two Aleve twice a day."

"Yes."

"It will diminish the inflammation. Hopefully you'll have less of these urinary symptoms."

"Okay."

"What I would do is stay on that for a month. And that's when you'll run out of Cardura. Stop that and stay on the Aleve."

"Okay."

"And see what happens to your urinary stream. If your urinary stream starts plugging up, then we'll have to put you on the Cardura for a little longer."

"Yes."

"But oftentimes a month is enough. Stay on the Aleve for a couple more weeks, then stop that. If you're feeling okay, you don't need either of them."

"Okay."

"I wouldn't stop them both together, because you wouldn't know which one . . . "

"Yes, I understand."

"Okay, let me tell you about the sex deal. When you have intercourse with ejaculation, you may have some pain. Because the prostate's contracting, and there's inflammation. You also may have some blood in the ejaculant. You should be forewarned."

"I had that after the biopsy."

"Right. For the first two weeks, you should use a condom, because sometimes a seed can come out."

"You've told us about that."

"Okay. I've told you this already. After that the seeds are going to stay pretty much where they are, and you don't need to worry."

"Good."

"I can't tell you whether the Cardura will effect your ability to have an erection. If it does, and it's a big issue, you can stop it sooner than a month."

"Right."

"Then see how your urinary flow is."

"Depending on that. On that list of medications, will you check off the ones you want me on?" Bob said.

"Yes. Right now. I'm supposed to do that."

"Okay, because I may not remember all of that."

"Yes. I wrote you an order."

"Do we come here tomorrow or to the hospital?" I asked.

"They should have something that tells you where the CT scan is being done. Let me look."

"And the chest X-ray," I added.

"Yes. Usually, we do them here. And I assume that CT scan is working at the moment. We have two CT scans. They'll tell you where to go."

"All right," Bob said.

"Get the CT scan. And then, if you have more questions, you can come by my office at the Northwest Tumor Institute."

"The radiation, I-125," Bob said.

"Yes?"

"When is it essentially 100% gone?"

"Technically never. But after six months, it has gone through three half-lives. The vast majority of it is gone. At that point, I would not worry about the radiation precautions."

"Okay. And the urethritis? How long will that last?"

Urethritis is inflammation of that part of the urethra that goes through the prostate gland and has been affected by the radiation.

"It can last anywhere from a few weeks to a few months. I've seen patients who still have urethritis nine months later. That's uncommon, but it can happen. My guess is that it will be most prominent between one week and four weeks. Then it will gradually subside over several weeks to several months."

"Okay."

"So we're giving you Bactrim, an antibiotic. We're giving you Cardura to help you void. I'm giving you some Tylenol #3 for pain. If the Aleve is not adequate in relieving discomfort, use the Tylenol, too. And the other thing we're giving you is a prescription for Pyridium."

"It makes you pee orange." I said.

"Yes, and it anesthetizes the bladder. Use it as needed."

"Bob can't write prescriptions here," I said.

"If you need a prescription, call me, and I'll take care of it."

"I have to go to the pharmacy for the medications. Right?"

"With my credit card, they can bill us and send them here," I said.

"We can do that. I think we talked earlier about radiation precautions—being careful around infants and pregnant women. In six months, you can forget about that. It doesn't matter with adults."

"I can hug him in the front, but I can't hug him in the back," I said.

"You can hug him anywhere you want."

"That's what I want to do," I said, still afraid of hurting him.

"Any other questions?"

"I think that pretty well covers it," Bob said and sounded worn out.

"So I think we're set," Dr. Meier said.

"Okay," we said in unison.

"You know, they've been going over today for their X-rays," I said.

"I'll have to see when yours is scheduled," a nurse walked in and said.

"We like to get them within 24 hours," Dr. Meier told her.

She looked at a chart.

"It's being done today on only the first two patients," she said. "So it will be tomorrow. I'll find out what time."

"Okay. If you have questions, you can come by tomorrow, but you don't have to," Dr. Meier said.

"All right," Bob said. "Thank you for all the care."

"You're welcome. It's been a pleasure to work with you."

"A pleasure?" I asked. "May I hug you?"

He laughed and said, "Absolutely. I'm not radioactive."

BOB

"Hey, look," I said. "My legs."

"Oh, good."

"Dr. Ragde and Dr. Meier to room 2, please," the intercom announced. "Dr. Ragde and Dr. Meier to room 2."

"Another one," I said.

The nurse came back and said, "10:45 tomorrow morning."

"Here, in this building?"

"Yes. Suite 130. And they usually like you to be here a little bit early. So be here at 10:30."

I was relieved that I didn't have anything else scheduled for today. I was bushed.

"If you'd like to have your prescriptions filled, I can fax them over to the pharmacy. They'll get them ready and send them over to you."

"Great."

A new nurse came in and said, "I'm going to take over while your nurse goes to lunch. How are your feet feeling?"

"Pretty normal, but not quite."

"A little bit tingly still?"

"Yes. A little."

"Okay. Have you ever had a spinal anesthetic before?"

"No."

"It wears off down the front. It spreads out over your toes, the soles of your feet. Then it wears off up the back of your legs. And your bottom is going to be the last spot to wear off."

She touched my foot and asked, "Does it feels a little like jello there?"

"It does. I'm getting there."

"Take your time," Saralee said.

"Is the IV still running?"

"Yes."

Saralee touched my left hand, near the IV insert tube. It was the first time she had touched me since surgery. It felt wonderful. I love having her near me.

"When the nurse sits me up, maybe she'll take the IV out."

"Maybe so. Don't rush things," Saralee said.

"Can I have another sandwich and another orange juice?" I asked my new nurse.

"I can get you another orange juice. We only order enough for each patient to have one sandwich."

"But there's a stack of sandwiches in the TV room," Saralee said.

"They're for the physicians who've come for the course."

"All right."

"I'll take a look, and if there are extras after they've left, I'll be happy to bring you one."

"Okay," I said, but I wanted the sandwich as ballast for my legs.

"Would you like another warm blanket?"

"No, I'm fine."

"Do you have an ice pack on?"

"Yes. They put one on. I can't feel it."

"You can't feel it yet?"

"It's there," I said and touched it with my free right hand. "It's kind of warm."

"I'll get you fresh ice."

I handed my ice pack to her, and she left my cubicle.

"It's warm?" Saralee asked.

"Oh, I don't know what's warm down there."

"Not an ice pack. That's you, baby."

The nurse came back with my refilled ice pack and said, "I'm going to turn you back over to your regular nurse. I'm going to lunch."

"Have a good lunch," I said. "We'll probably be gone when you get back here."

I certainly hoped so. I wanted to get up, to get moving.

"Oh, there's Dr. Ragde," Saralee said. "I want to hug him again."

She went to Dr. Ragde, and I heard him ask. "It's all good?"

Saralee returned elated and said, "It's done. It's really done."

"Yes, the procedure is done. It's over. I'm so close, but not quite yet."

"Hey, take your time. We've got tons of time. Together time."

Shannon came in and said, "Would you like to try sitting up?"

"Sure," I said.

"Do it slowly."

I did as told and found it difficult because of the additional pressure on my perineum.

"I want to try to urinate," I said.

"Great," she said. "I'll disconnect your IV first."

She slid it out painlessly.

"The bathroom is down the hall next to the changing room. Do you need help getting there?"

I stood up to test my legs and said, "I don't think so."

I shuffled to the bathroom in my paper slippers. I stood over the toilet for a while, but I couldn't make it happen. I shuffled back to my cubicle and reclining chair. I wanted to lie down but resisted the temptation.

"Any luck?" Shannon asked.

"No," I said, dejected.

"I'll get you some more juice."

"It's okay," Saralee said. "Be patient."

Saralee was well aware that patience is not one of my virtues. I drank the juice quickly. I'd lost count of how many cans I'd drunk since surgery. If I could walk and urinate, they'd release me.

A woman came with a bag containing my medications.

"I have a charge card to pay for them," Saralee said.

"That's not necessary. We'll bill you for them."

"Thanks," I said.

"I'll hold onto that for you," Saralee said and put the medicines in the plastic bag with my clothes.

"I think I'll try to urinate again."

"Do you feel the need to tinkle?"

"I think so."

I was successful. I came back with a smile plastered on my face.

"You did it, baby."

"Right. When can we leave?"

Shannon had followed me into my cubicle and overheard me.

"Anytime you want. Is your car far from the entrance?"

"We didn't come by car. We came by taxi."

"I have a whole list of radio cabs," Saralee said and fished through her purse for them.

"I don't need them," Shannon said. "I'll be able to get you a taxi."

She handed me a wet cloth and said, "This is to help you wipe off the Betadine."

"Thanks."

"Here's a pad to put inside your jockey shorts in case you bleed. Do you need help dressing?" Shannon asked.

"Certainly not."

Shannon pulled the curtain around the front of my recovery area.

The curtain had been pulled along the sides but not across the front until now. I used the wet cloth and reached for the bag with my clothes.

"Wait a minute," Saralee said. "You still have Betadine on your back. Let me wipe it off."

When she had finished, I dressed myself and sat down again in my chair, surprised that such a simple act could be so tiring.

Shannon returned and called through the curtain, "Are you dressed yet?"

"Definitely," I said with pride.

She opened the curtain and said, "Here is an empty ice pack to use when you get back to the hotel."

"Thanks."

"And a strainer for your urine. Use the strainer until you come back tomorrow. If you find a radioactive seed in the strainer, pick it up with this tweezers and put it in this container. Bring it back to us. I've called for your cab."

"Thanks."

"There's a personnel room beside the door. It has an exit of its own. You'll be more comfortable waiting there."

"Thanks again."

"Yes. Good luck."

She directed us to the personnel room. It had chairs, but I was more comfortable standing. The cab came soon.

The ride back was uncomfortable. The driver said he had over 100,000 miles on his taxi. The lumpy seat attested to that.

I couldn't sit flat and rotated from one buttock to the other. When we turned corners, I was thrown off balance. The driver kept talking, and I was in no mood for conversation. All I wanted was my bed.

Finally in our room, I poured a glass of water and took Bactrim, my antibiotic, and two Aleves and a Tylenol for pain. I undressed and checked my pad. It had pinpoints of blood on it. I got into pajamas.

Saralee folded back the bedspread and said, "I'll fill your ice pack."

She looked through the plastic bag but couldn't find the ice pack they had given me. Neither could I. I wanted to get into bed, to go to sleep. I gave Saralee a face towel from the bathroom.

"Let's use this as a substitute," I said. "Put ice in the plastic bag and cover it with the towel."

She pulled back the covers on my side of the bed and got the ice.

I positioned the "ice pack" on my perineum and fell sound asleep. I woke up at dusk. Saralee sat on our sofa with an open book on her lap and looked at me.

"Why aren't you reading?" I asked.

"Because I'd rather look at you. May I sit on the bed beside you?"

"Of course."

She sat beside me and held my hand.

"Your fingers feel so warm and cozy," she said. "You have immaculate hands."

"Thanks," I said. "Your fingers feel cool and comforting."

"I want to hold you in my arms, but I'm afraid that might hurt you."

"I understand."

We held hands and watched dusk turn into night.

"What time is it?" I asked.

She told me that it was past 6 P.M. I was surprised that I had slept so long.

"How do you feel?" she asked.

"Sore, tired."

"We have a dinner reservation at Tulio's downstairs," she said, "but I have a better idea."

"What's that?"

"Tulio's does room service. We could drink our own wine instead of theirs. We have too much wine."

"Whose fault is that?"

"I refuse to answer. I'm pleading the fifth."

She handed me the menu and said, "Start choosing."

We each chose. She phoned the order and canceled our reservation at the restaurant.

"Do you want a glass of wine or would you rather stick to water?" she asked.

"Water first, wine afterwards."

I drank the water quickly. She poured me a glass of wine. We sipped wine companionably until dinner arrived. The food tasted wonderful—the first real meal since breakfast yesterday. Saralee's risotto with scallops, leeks, and saffron butter smelled delicious, and I ploughed through a bowl of minestrone followed by a chicken breast topped with carmelized garlic and served with lemon risotto. I fell asleep soon after dinner.

My penis and scrotum were both swollen and blood engorged the next morning. My perineum was sore. Other than that, I felt pretty good.

A drop of my blood had spilled onto the bathroom floor. I cleaned it up fast, before Saralee could see it. She's squeamish about blood.

Saralee showed me a stain on her right hand, left over from wiping off my Betadine, and I said, "A last memento of surgery."

We arrived at the outpatient clinic early, so I had my chest X-ray before the CT scan. I waited for the film to be processed, and read it. There were no seeds in my chest. I told the technician not to bill me for a professional fee, because I had interpreted the film myself. She looked at me as if I were crazy.

SARALEE

We went to Suite 130 for Bob's CT scan. He had told me that the scan bisects the prostate gland every 5 millimeters and provides multiple images.

Bob lowered his pants and was positioned on a flat table which would put all of his anatomy at the same perspective. The technician tied his feet together with a rubber cord. He put a rubber pad under Bob's back for support on the flat table and a towel under Bob's knees to lessen the strain on his back.

He slid Bob into a gantry, an enclosure larger than an MRI and less claustrophobic. Bob was tilted at a 15-degree angle so the gantry wouldn't be close to his face. The technician and I went into the next room where the CT-scan images would be projected on a screen. A glass wall separated us from Bob.

Sliver after sliver of Bob's prostate shone on the screen. Each glowed with lights of radioactive seeds, the sparkling lights of health. I found myself drawn into the luminous field. I skimmed between and sailed beside stars—afloat. His prostate had been transformed to a starry sky.

Healing

⁓

Bob's body healed rapidly, so much so that he needed to use the condoms he had stocked beforehand. His first ejaculation was painful and bloody, as Dr. Meier had predicted. Several others were blood-tinged, but painless and meaningful for both of us. We remain happy bunnies in bed.

Bob did not take the prescribed Cardura for fear it would cause impotence. His urethra blocked several weeks after surgery, and his local urologist catherized him for four days. Following the removal of the catheter, he had no further urine-retention problems. In retrospect, he realized that we should have followed Dr. Meier's advice about Cardura.

Six weeks after surgery Bob's PSA was 4.04, higher than before surgery. Frightened, he called Dr. Ragde, who suspected a prostate infection due to post-surgical inflammation and prescribed Cipro, an antibiotic. Bob's PSA descended as the radioactive pellets did their job to 1.81 in March and 1.36 in May.

For a month or two after surgery Bob experienced the anticipated burning sensation while urinating. The anticipated urgency, frequency, and diminished stream lingered for several more months. They're now gone.

The emotional scars that affirmed our vulnerability during the first several months after surgery amazed us both. We experienced more fear and expressed more anger than we did when confronting Bob's disease, because cancer had shattered the illusion that he controls his life. We had promised each other a normal life after surgery, and nothing felt normal after the trauma we had survived.

Transcendent images remained then—Mt. Rainier, Haakon Ragde, a prostate turned starry sky, and Bob, who cooked dinner occasionally while Saralee chose and sampled the wine. Viva.

Bob retired from his country hospital on his sixty-sixth birthday. Healed, happy, and relaxed now, he's expanding his skills in cooking, tennis, bridge, and investments. After an orientation about the visually impaired, he was assigned Jeff, a blind attorney, whose only need is to be taken shopping at the local A & P. The two men usually shop together on a weekend morning. Bob brings home a few groceries for us, too.

Bob is writing literary criticism about Henry James's *The American* for a course he's taking in American literature at a local college, while Saralee pecks out our epilogue. This is the second literature course he has taken. He enjoys delving into the layers of meaning in a book and writes better literary criticism than I ever wrote.

When not at work writing our book, I occasionally remember to send out poems for publication. Three new poems have been accepted by *Parnassus Literary Journal.*

In April 1998, Dr. Haakon Ragde published his ten-year disease-free statistics for early stage, gland confined treatment of prostate cancer with ultrasound-guided radioactive seed implants at 66%. Published 10-year statistics for radical prostatectomy range mainly from 47% to 73%. A PSA of 0.5 or lower is a standard of measurement.

Bob's PSA jumped from 1.36 to 2.29 in August. Neither Dr. Ragde nor Dr. Meier was available on the Friday afternoon he got the test results. And Bob's local urologist had left his office for the day. Bob spoke with a local pathologist who told him that the upsurge in PSA meant a recurrence of cancer. I kept us very busy that weekend to mask our fear.

We saw Bob's local urologist on Monday morning. He examined Bob and told him that his prostate was flat as a pancake, the desired effect. He claimed that PSA stood for "patient-stimulated anxiety."

Bob spoke with Dr. Meier and Dr. Ragde on Monday afternoon. Dr. Meier faxed him a medical article that showed a benign upsurge in PSA between 12 and 24 months after I-125 implantation in a third of the cases. The article indicated that when PSA rises instead of falling, the patient panics, a truth to which we can attest. Dr. Ragde prescribed an antibiotic in case some infection had occurred.

Bob's next PSA in November had dropped to 1.05. We feel certain that it will drop to 0.5 in the projected 18 to 24 months following I-125 implants.

We have ascended beyond fear and anger now and spend little time worrying about prostate cancer or lupus. We believe they're both past tense. Our life together is blessedly normal—except for one vast difference. Everything we share has increased meaning. It's always a beautiful day.

Afterword

BY

HAAKON RAGDE, M.D., F.A.C.S.

~

Dear Friends,

I think you have done a wonderful job by producing something that has never been done before to my knowledge. It certainly brings home the emotional aspect when one is confronted with cancer close to home and also the confusing aspect of the treatment recommendations. The latter is particularly impressive—when even someone with medical training becomes confused.

When you, Bob, say, "I'm all mixed up as to what therapy to have," that tells it all. One wonders how confused someone without any medical training would be. The moment one wanders beyond the primary diagnosis of the disease and attempts to decide what treatment is appropriate for him, a sense of bewilderment and disorientation occurs. Until this investitgative patient decides for himself, his life lacks focus and order.

Your description of the emotional ups and downs when confronted with a diagnosis of prostate cancer in a family member is good, Saralee. It brought me back to the spring of 1963 when I was given a diagnosis of fibrosarcoma of my right arm, arising from the scar of one of my shrapnel wounds suffered in Korea. It was a terrible two weeks while I debated with myself whether or not I should allow them to disarticulate the arm at the shoulder. Had the disease already spread elsewhere?

I finally asked for a second opinion from the pathology department at the Sloan Kettering Cancer Center in New York. A few days later, I was told the lesion was benign. They called it "sclerosing adenitis." A few years ago, they said, they would also have labeled it a fibrosarcoma and recommended surgical removal.

I know you consider yourself a well man, Bob, and rightfully so. Please keep in touch with me, Saralee, and let me know how and what both of you are doing.

Sincerely,

Haakon

Resources

~

There are numerous treatment options, especially if the cancer is caught early and tests indicate a likelihood of confinement to the gland. Chances are the patient will have to decide his treatment, and will be confused. The first thing we advise reading is Andy Grove's article "Taking on Prostate Cancer" in the May 13, 1996, issue of *Fortune* magazine. He thought it through for himself, and so can others.

Then, it would be helpful to consult the American Cancer Society's *Prostate Cancer, What Every Man—and His Family—Needs to Know,* by David G. Bostwick, M.D., Gregory T. MacLennan, M.D., and Thayne R. Larson, M.D., New York: Random House, 1996.

For an account of radical prostatectomy and its aftermath, done by a widely respected surgeon, Dr. Patrick Walsh at Johns Hopkins in Baltimore, one should read Michael Korda's *Man to Man: Surviving Prostate Cancer,* New York: Random House, 1996.

ADDITIONAL BOOKS YOU MAY WANT TO READ:

Goldenberg, S. Larry. *All You Need to Know to Take an Active Part in Your Treatment, 2nd edition.* New York: Houghton Mifflin, 1997.

Hitchcox, Robert. *Love, Sex and PSA: Living and Loving With Prostate Cancer.* San Diego, California: TNC Press, 1997.

Kaltenbach, Don and Tim Richards. *Prostate Cancer: A Survivor's Guide.* New Port Richey, Florida: Seneca House Press, 1995.

Kantoff, Phillip, M.D. with Malcolm McConnell. *Prostate Cancer: A Family Consultation.* New York: Houghton-Mifflin, 1996.

Lewis, James, Jr., Ph.D. And E. Roy Berger, M.D. *New Guidelines for Surviving Prostate Cancer.* Westbury, New York. Health Education Literary Publisher, 1997.

Loo, Marcus H. and Marian Betancourt. *The Prostate Cancer Sourcebook: How to Make Informed Treatment Choices.* New York: John Wiley and Sons, 1998.

Maddox, Robert. *Prostate Cancer: What I found Out and What You Should Know.* Wheaton, Illinois: Harold Shaw Publishers, 1997.

Marks, Sheldon, M.D. *Prostate and Cancer: A Family Guide to Diagnosis, Treatment, and Survival.* Tucson: Fisher Books, 1995.

Meyer, Sylvan, and Seymour C. Nash, M.D. *Prostate Cancer, Making Survival Decisions.* Chicago: The University of Chicago Press, 1994.

Morra, Marion E., et al. *The Prostate Cancer Answer Book: A Guide to Treatment Choices.* New York: Avon Books, 1996.

Osterling, Joseph E. and Mark A. Movad. *The A B C's of Prostate Cancer: The Book That Could Save Your Life.* Lanham, Maryland: Madison Books, 1997.

Payne, James E. *Me Too: A Doctor Survives Prostate Cancer.* Waco, Texas: WRS Publishing, 1995.

Phillips, Robert H., Ph.D. *Coping With Prostate Cancer.* Garden City Park, New York: Avery Publishing Group, 1994.

Salowe, Allen E. *Prostate Cancer: Overcoming Denial With Action: A Guide to Screening, Treatment, and Healing.* New York: St. Martin's Griffin, 1998.

Wainrib, Barbara Rubin, et al. *Prostate Cancer: A Guide for Women and the Men They Love.* New York: Dell Books, 1996.

Walsh, Patrick C., M.D. and Janet Farrar Worthington. *The Prostate: A Guide for Men and the Women Who Love Them.* Baltimore: The Johns Hopkins Press, 1995. (Dr. Walsh was Michael Korda's surgeon.)

Support Organizations to Contact

Ablin Foundation for Cancer Research
115 Franklin Turnpike, Suite 200
Mahwah, New Jersey 07430
Develops and improves methods of early detection, diagnosis, and treatment of prostate cancer.

American Cancer Society
1599 Clifton Road, NE
Atlanta, Georgia 30329
800-227-2345
This is a most comprehensive source for all cancer information. It provides literature, sponsors support groups, cancer recovery programs, and funds research. It is the national base for Man to Man, support groups for men who have or have had prostate cancer in numerous communities across the U.S. and for Side by Side for couples.

American Foundation for Urologic Disease
1126 North Charles Street
Baltimore, Maryland 21201
410-468-1800
Information for patients and professionals about prostate cancer and impotence.

The American Prostate Society
1340F Charwood Road
Hanover, Maryland 21076
410-859-3735
Dedicated to early detection and treatment of prostate cancer, thereby cutting deaths by 50%.

American Psychiatric Association
Division of Public Affairs, Dept. ACS
1400 K Street, NW
Washington, DC 20005
202-682-6325
How to cope with anxiety, depression, and other psychological side effects.

American Urological Association
1120 North Charles Street
Baltimore, Maryland 21201
410-223-4310
Information for patients and professionals, research and education.

Canadian Cancer Society
10 Alcorn Acorn Avenue, Suite 200
Toronto, Ontario
Canada M4V 3B1
416-961-7223
Canada's equivalent to the American Cancer Society.

Cancer Care, Inc.
1180 Avenue of the Americas
New York, New York 10036
800-813-4673 and 212-221-3300
Informs and counsels patients and their families.

Cancer Hot Line
4410 Main Street
Kansas City, Missouri 64111
816-932-8453
Information, referrals, and books for patients and their families.

Cancer Support Network
5895 Devereau Lane
Pittsburgh, Pennsylvania 15232
412-661-8949
Workshops and support groups for patients and families.

CaP CURE
1250 Fourth Street, Suite 360
Santa Monica, California 90401
310-458-2873
Michael Milken's organization seeking a cure for prostate cancer.

First Call for Help
United Way of Southwestern Indiana
812-421-2800
Mutual and community support groups for prostate cancer.

International Isotopes, Inc.
3100 Jim Christal Road
Denton Texas 76207
940-484-9492
The newest kid on the block who will begin producing radioactive isotopes in 1999, including those used in treating prostate cancer.

Impotence World Institute
PO Box 410
Bowie, Maryland 20718
800-669-1603
Offers Impotence Anonymous support groups.

The Mathews Foundation for Prostate Cancer Research
817 Common Drive
Sacramento, California 95825
800-234-6284
Telephone counseling, books, videotapes, research funds.

National Association for Continence
PO Box 8310
Spartanburg, South Carolina 29305
800-252-3337
Newsletter, informative guide, and physician referral for incontinence.

National Cancer Institute
National Institute of Health Building 31, Room 10A24
Bethesda, Maryland 20814
800-422-6237
Information about cancer treatment, care centers, and research for patients and professionals that is government sponsored.

National Chronic Pain Outreach Association
7979 Old Georgetown Road, Suite 100
Bethesda, Maryland 20814
301-652-4948
Free brochure about dealing with pain.

National Coalition for Cancer Survivorship
1010 Wayne Avenue, Fifth Floor
Silver Springs, Maryland 20910
301-650-8868
Survivors network that provides support group information and stresses rights of cancer patients.

National Prostate Cancer Coalition
1156 15th Street, Suite 905
Washington, DC 20005
202-463-9455
Dedicated to bringing together organizations and individuals interested in prevention and cure of prostate cancer. Not a support group, but most support groups are represented in the coalition.

Nycomed Amersham/Nycomed Amersham Imaging
110 Carnegie Center
Princeton, New Jersey 08450-6231
609-514-6000
Producers of Iodine-125 radioactive seeds.

Patient Advocates for Advanced Cancer Treatments
1143 Parmelee, NW
Grand Rapids, Michigan 49504
616-453-1477
Nonprofit support of hormone use, cryosurgery, and other alternative treatments.

Prostate Cancer Research Network
PO Box 966
Port Richey, Florida 34656
813-847-1619
Designed to help those faced with prostate cancer.

Prostate Cancer Support Network
1218 North Charles Street
Baltimore, Maryland 21201
800-828-7866
Affiliate of the American Foundation for Urologic Disease that focuses public attention on evaluation and treatment of patients.

Prostate Information Hotline
800-543-9632
Information service regarding prostate cancer.

SEICUS (Sexual Information and Education Council of the United States)
130 West 42nd Street
New York, New York 10036
212-819-9770
Focuses on incontinence treatment.

The Simon Foundation
PO Box 835
Wilmette, Illinois 60091
800-237-4666
Education regarding incontinence treatment.

Theragenics Corporation
5325 Oak Brook Parkway
Norcross, Georgia 30093
800-458-4372
Information about radiation seed implantation using Palladium-103.

US TOO International, Inc.
930 North York Road, Suite 50
Hinsdale, Illinois 60521
800-808-7866
Nationwide list of over 900 organizations for people afflicted by diseases. Lists organizations by disease names. Especially interested in prostate cancer with local chapters all across the United States.

Women's Suffrage for Prostate Cancer Awareness and Support
733 Caribou Court
Sunnyvale, California 94087
888-776-2262
Support for cancer victims' female partners.

Computer-Based Resources

According to our local newspaper, professional matchmakers have been replaced by cyber-courting. The world-wide web can help you learn about prostate cancer and participate in decision making. Here are a few web sites to begin your search for well-being.

American Cancer Society
http://www.cancer.org/

American Foundation for Urologic Disease
http://www.afud.org

Cancer Care, Inc.
http://www.cancercare.org

National Association for Continence
http://www.nafc.org

Northwest Hospital
http://nwhospital.org

Prostate Cancer InfoLink
http://www.comed.com.Prostate/

If the web site address has changed, type in the name of the organization instead.

Cruising the web is wonderful sport. One site leads to another. If you can't find a specific site on Yahoo, switch to Alta Vista or another search engine. The web expands so rapidly that new sites appear daily, and old ones disappear. Bulletin boards and chat groups exist.

You can also get information by typing in a topic, such as prostate cancer, on the search option. You're the boss.

Index

~